ULTIMATE Pilates

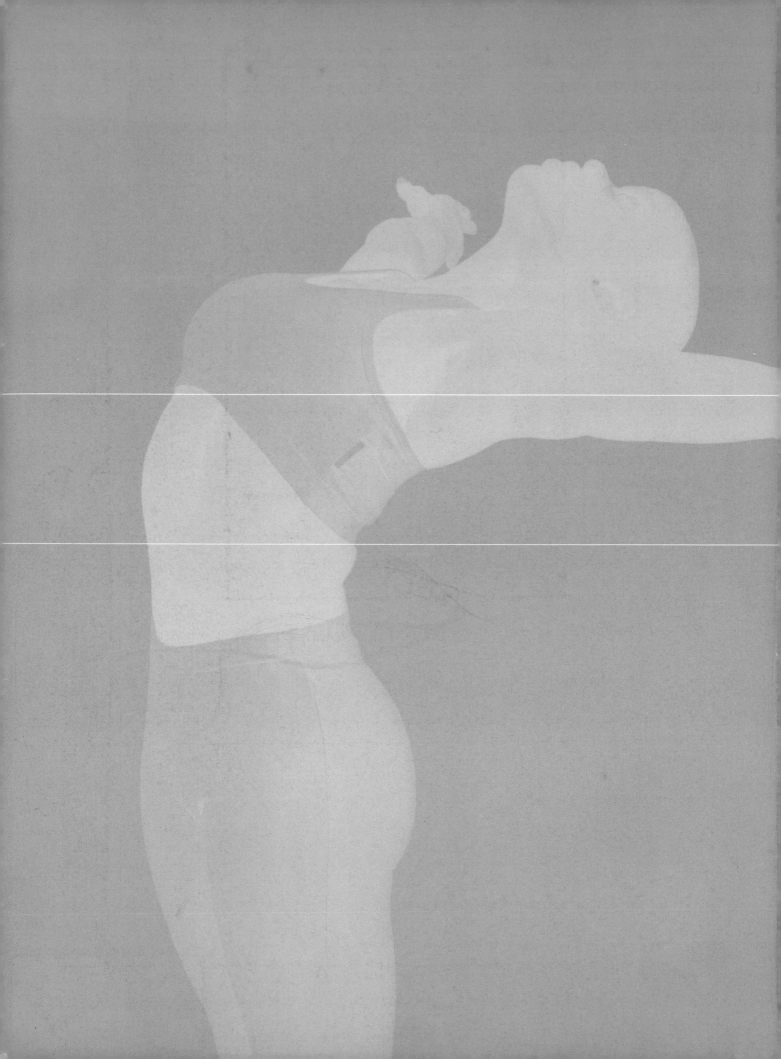

ULTIMATE
Pilates

Dreas Reyneke

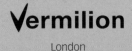

Vermilion

London

Dedication

to Janine Ulfane
and for all my pupils

First published in Great Britain in 2002 by Ebury Press,
an imprint of Random House,
20 Vauxhall Bridge Road, London SW1V 2SA

Random House Australia (Pty) Limited
20 Alfred Street, Milson's Point, Sydney,
New South Wales 2061, Australia

Random House New Zealand Limited
18 Poland Road, Glenfield, Auckland 10,
New Zealand

Random House South Africa (Pty) Limited
Endulin, 5A Jubilee Road, Parktown 2193,
South Africa

The Random House Group Limited Reg. No. 954009

www.randomhouse.co.uk

A CIP catalogue record for this book is available from the British Library.

Design: The Design Revolution Ltd
1st Floor, Queens Park Villa, 30 West Drive,
Brighton, East Sussex BN2 0QW, UK

Special photography by Steve Gorton

Illustrations:
Gill Oliver; Halli Verrinder

Picture research:
Penni Bickle Research

ISBN 0091876710

Papers used by Ebury Press are natural, recyclable products made from wood grown in sustainable forests.

Printed in Germany

**If you have a medical condition, or are
pregnant, the exercises described in this book
should not be followed without first consulting
your doctor. All guidelines and warnings should
be read carefully and the author and publishers
cannot accept responsibility for injuries or damage
arising out of a failure to comply with the same.**

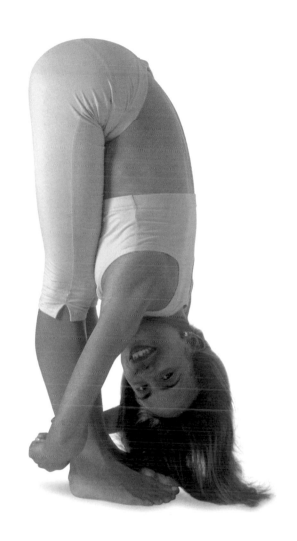

Dreas teaching structural pilates:
It's like you were once a VW bus and then
you're a Ferrari. My husband thanks you.

RUBY WAX, TV INTERVIEWER, COMEDIENNE, AND ONE-WOMAN STAGE ENTERTAINER

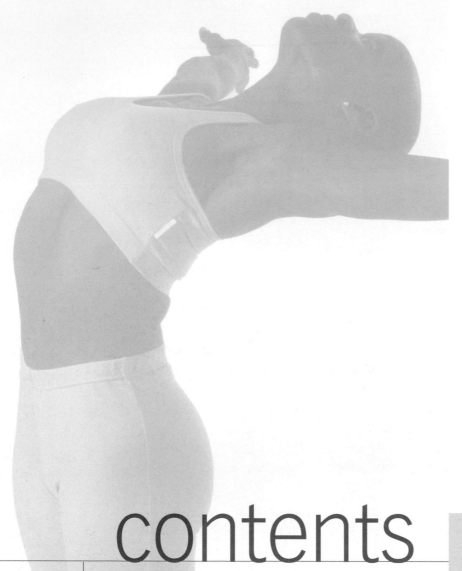

contents

Once I was bent. Now I'm straight. Dreas
has taught me to stretch and strengthen my
body – in terms that my non-physical mind
can comprehend. As a result, all aspects of
my life have improved.

MARTIN SHERMAN, PLAYWRIGHT

Preface

My long association with pilates began in London during the 1960s, when, as a dancer with the Ballet Rambert I found pilates stretches essential for all-round fitness, a fantastic supplement to dance exercises. Each day before practice I would work on my body structure, balance, and symmetry. I learned the classic pilates system taught by people who had studied in New York under former students of the founder of the pilates system, Joseph Hubertus Pilates.

Joseph Pilates was a fitness instructor who emigrated to the USA from Germany in 1923. In the early years of the 20th century most exercise regimes worked at building and strengthening muscles by repetitive exercises such as press-ups, push-ups, and weightlifting. Pilates' approach was holistic, based on toning the body and correcting poor posture with progressively more difficult exercises carried out slowly and with concentration, involving mind as well as body.

Professional dancers were enthusiastic regulars at Pilates' New York studio during the 1950s and 1960s. No doubt they found his exercises helped correct the postural defects and heal the whole-body effects of the injuries they suffered in performance. When I retired from dancing I taught at the first pilates studio in London, at The Place, the home of contemporary dance in London. I found myself interpreting Pilates' teachings to a new generation of dancers and discovered that my background and understanding gave me a different slant on them. Wanting to explore this pathway, I opened my studio in London's Notting Hill in 1973, and there I reviewed Pilates' teachings, and brought to them a new perspective.

Every body has a unique structure, every mind is different, and everyone brings to my studio a unique set of requirements and an individual approach to the exercises. My clients have been the main impetus behind my interpretation of Joseph Pilates' system. Some studios try to make everyone do the same exercises in the same rigidly disciplined way, but this is to distort the body into the shape of the exercise system. We all need to be more conscious of how dependent we are on our marvellous bodies. I once taught children handicapped by polio and birth defects, and I saw what extraordinary achievements a body can make if it can be approached in a way to which it is able to respond. Working with my clients, who are people from diverse professions and backgrounds, of all ages, with wide-ranging needs and expectations, I listen to the needs of each individual's body and mind, and adapt the exercises to meet them.

Clients from many major international dance companies have been a source of inspiration. They contribute unusual problems, and solving them generates new ideas. Searching for ways to help them heal their injuries and achieve their goals, I explored the ideas of the American physiologist and biochemist Ida Rolf, whose seminal work during the 1960s on the structural role of the connective tissues is now widely known and respected. People are generally unaware of imbalances in their body structure, and I sought ways of analyzing each individual's needs, from toe to head.

Physical and mental tension are universal 21st-century experiences. They are the cause of much unhappiness and illness which many therapists have sought to alleviate. During my teaching career, I returned to study. For three years I learned shiatsu massage under a Japanese teacher in London, Uichi Kawada, and part of my approach to exercise is to use massage as a sure way of relieving physical and mental tension at the end or at the beginning of a session.

Teachers need to learn from their students, and I became aware of the role of breathing in stress management and structural fitness from teachers of Alexander Technique who visited my studio. Through them I understood how tension can inhibit breathing. They also led me to explore the link between the diaphragm and the internal muscles in the lower part of the abdomen – the pelvic floor.

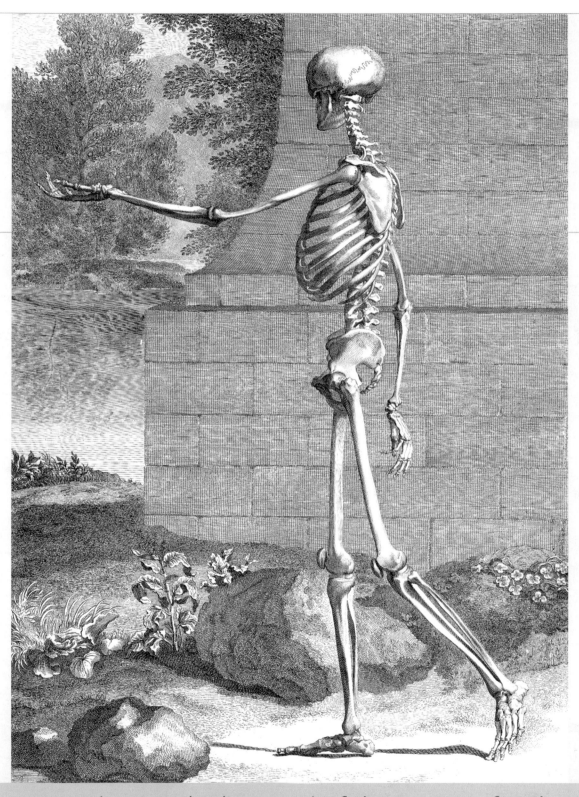

Joseph Pilates may have admired the perfect posture of this Male skeleton seen from the side. It was one of four plates engraved by Simon François Ravenet the elder to illustrate an anatomy book, Tabulae squeletare et muscularum by B.S. Albinus, published in 1747.

Dreas understands the need of the non-professional body to find its own individual potential. SALLY POTTER, WRITER, ACTRESS, FILM DIRECTOR

Years ago I was introduced to the pioneering work of Peter Blythe and Sally Goddard at the Institute for Neuro-Physiological Psychology in the UK. Their studies of how infants learn to move, and how learning difficulties such as dyslexia may result if the natural learning process is inhibited in early life are now widely known, and they have resulted in new discoveries about movement patterns in adults. I found they illuminated problems of coordination and balance experienced by some of my clients and, as a result, I devised new ways of helping these clients overcome their difficulties of movement through exercise.

Rather than apply the pilates system rigidly, my aim has always been to help people overcome their problems, and this occasionally leads me into conflict with traditional pilates teaching. Many taboos about the body have been overcome since Pilates thought and taught. In 1968, for example, an American physician, Arnold Kegel, first publicized the importance of exercising

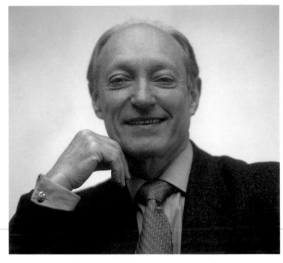

The exercises I present in this book are gentle and relaxing. If you practise them regularly and with concentration, they will tone your muscles, improve your posture, strengthen your whole body, relax and fortify your mind, and raise your spirits.

When I first went to Dreas I was the kind of 48-year-old who would groan every time he moved. Thanks to him I have stopped groaning. Dreas has a deep understanding of how the body works.

MARTIN AMIS, WRITER

the muscles of the pelvic floor. I see traditional pilates teachers emphasize the technique of pulling the navel back toward the spine to tone the abdominal muscles. But the navel-to-spine technique has the side effect of inhibiting breathing. Working on Kegel's observations, I emphasize lifting the pelvic floor, a technique that has immensely beneficial effects on posture, balance, stability, and mental wellbeing.

Like Joseph Pilates I teach one-to-one at my studio, so I can reach only a limited number of people. To try to reach and help a wider public I have devised a programme of exercises for people to practise alone at

home, and I present them in this book. If you follow the programme through, practising regularly with effort and dedication, the exercises will help you balance and restructure your body. You do not need to have attended pilates sessions in the past, and you need no special equipment. The only rule is that you must begin at the beginning and learn the exercises in sequence. The programme is planned first to address your body's structural problems and improve its posture, and then to integrate each change into your way of moving, so that it becomes a part of your natural movement pattern. This approach effects changes subtly with regular practice,

A lot of fun, and laughter. A plastic surgeon for the body, but without the plastic – or, indeed, the surgery.

HELENA BONHAM CARTER, FILM ACTRESS

and because of this you need to review your progress at regular intervals. To help you make regular reviews I have divided the programme into three levels, with a review session at the end of the first two – so on pages 138–39 and pages 170–71 you revisit and revise what you have learned. Doing this gives you a different perspective on each exercise, and it should open your mind and liberate your body to new movement experiences.

Make pilates exercise sessions a regular part of your life and you will improve your structural fitness and become generally healthier. Begin by striving to assess and understand your body's structural strengths and weaknesses (turn to Part 4 to find out how), and then work on overcoming its defects. And then you must continue, through exercise, to understand your body's changes, week by week, for the rest of your life.

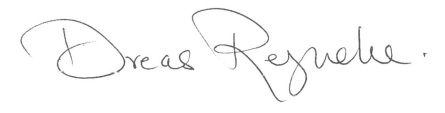

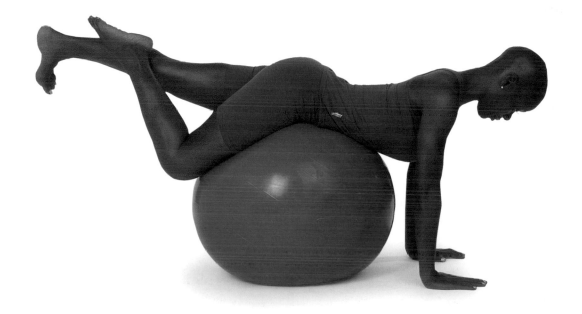

part 1
body-conditioning

Physical fitness is the first
requisite for happiness.

Joseph Pilates

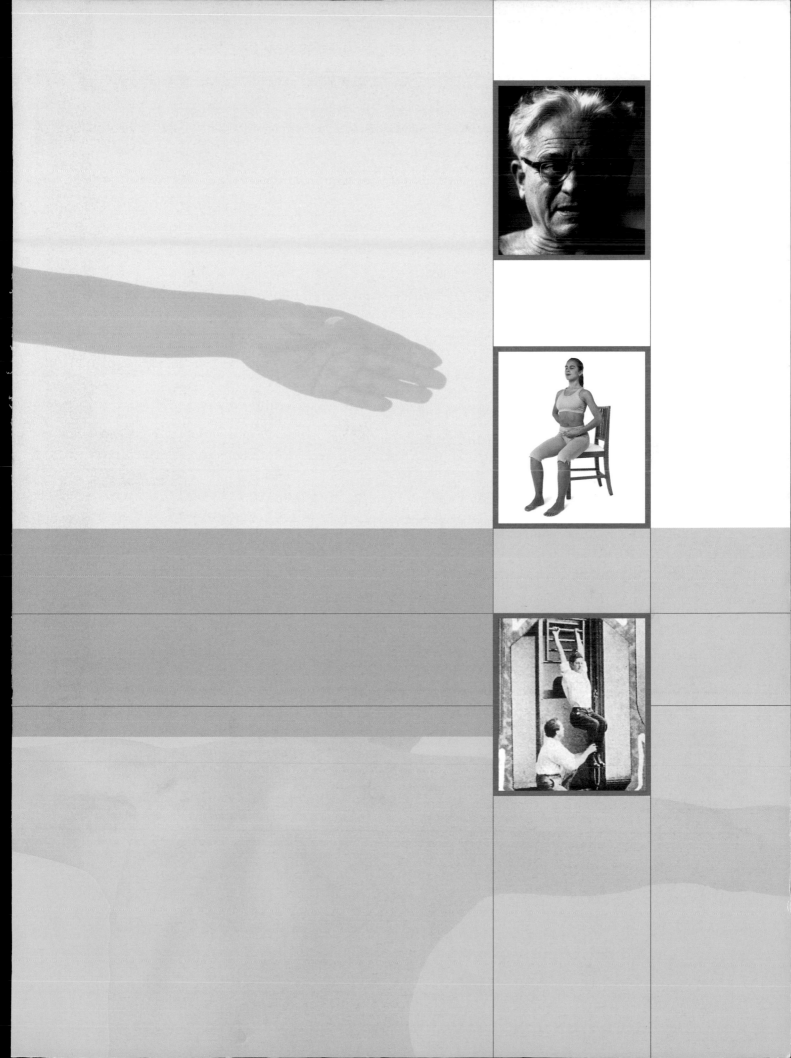

Why Pilates?

Back at the beginning of the 20th century Joseph Pilates warned of the ill effects of the fast tempo of modern living, and of the need to keep the body healthy and to develop the mind. In the 1920s he was already concerned with ways of combating unnatural physical fatigue and nervous strain caused by the use of telephones and automobiles, and by economic and political pressures. He published his exercises as a remedy for the effects of what we now call stress, and the results of physical neglect. By practising them, he believed, his clients could acquire control of the body and regain the natural rhythm and coordination of movement that civilized living erodes.

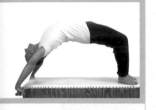

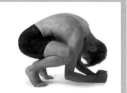

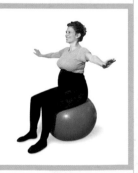

Pilates exercises are ideal for everyone from the late teens, all through adult life into extreme old age.

Rather than overdevelop certain muscles, as in weight-lifting or work exclusively on one part of the body, such as the hips and thighs, pilates stretches and exercises the whole body. Pilates teaches correct breathing, emphasizing rhythmic movements of the diaphragm – the large muscle whose actions force air in and out of the lungs – and prolonged, controlled out-breaths. Several classic pilates exercises involve gently rolling the spine down and then up, which exercises the lungs in addition to improving the spine's flexibility.

Joseph Pilates' original fitness programme consisted of 34 exercises, which, he declared, would transform the body if practised regularly. Although his successors have simplified these exercises into movement sequences more easily learned by beginners, we all teach fundamentally the same core exercises to the original timescale established by the founder.

My exercise programme in Part 5 expands the classic pilates repertoire to meet the needs of different people. Those in the late teens and early twenties often need to concentrate on improving overall coordination. Someone who has worked in the same profession for years might need to overcome a stoop or a left-right imbalance brought about by habits of standing or sitting at work. Mothers may need to restore the elasticity of the pelvic floor. And if you are in your later years, you will want to focus on maintaining the mobility of muscles and joints.

True to Joseph Pilates' principle of balancing body and mind, the programme begins with posture. The first exercises relax neck and shoulders to encourage the correct balance of head on spine. Many beginners are

surprised to find that positioning the head correctly increases the field of vision. Postural defects can encourage a habit of looking down, or even upward, or off to one side. The postural exercises on pages 62–65 and 95–99 level the head, so the eyes look straight ahead, taking more in and increasing awareness. Body posture takes its cue from the balance of the upper body, so holding the head upright and the shoulders down realigns the spine, allowing it to transmit the weight of the body to the hips and equally down both legs to the feet.

Whole-body exercise

What makes modern pilates different from some other ways of exercising is the way the exercises are performed. By contrast with the mindless repetitions of step aerobics or weight training, for example, pilates exercises require concentration and attention to detail: to the exact position of a foot or the arc of movement of a shoulder. The result is not to strengthen one muscle or one set of muscles, but to benefit the whole body. Exercising the muscles of the pelvic floor, for example, improves posture, relieves backache, and flattens the stomach.

The pilates-based exercises in this book are gentle and designed to be carried out slowly and rhythmically. If you practise with care and attention to the position and movement of your body parts, they will correct postural defects and improve the fitness of your whole body, inside and out and from head to toe. One immediate benefit is a sense of wellbeing. In time and with perseverance they will also condition your body, improving its appearance and its carriage and bearing.

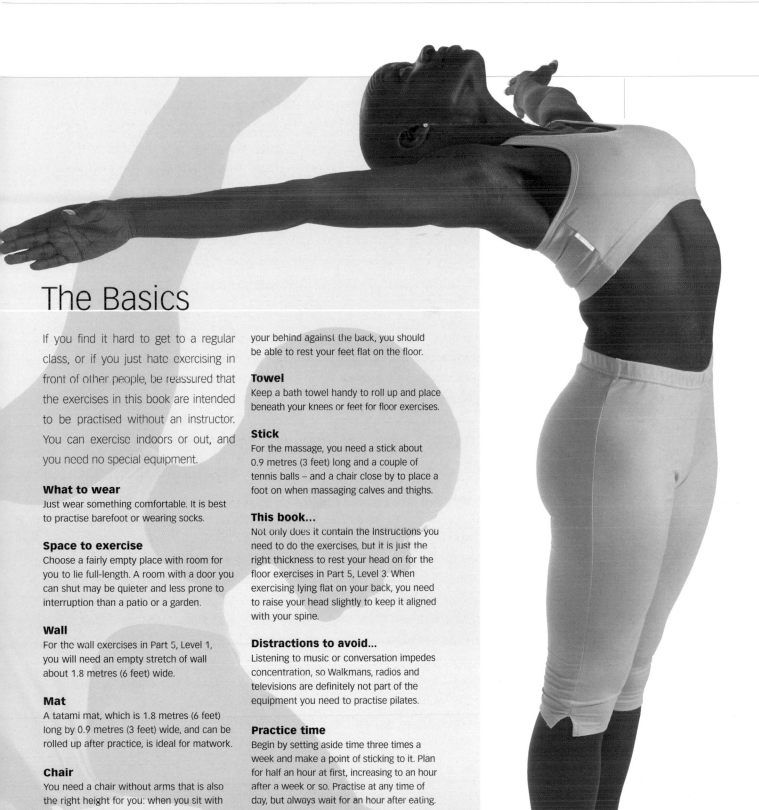

The Basics

If you find it hard to get to a regular class, or if you just hate exercising in front of other people, be reassured that the exercises in this book are intended to be practised without an instructor. You can exercise indoors or out, and you need no special equipment.

What to wear
Just wear something comfortable. It is best to practise barefoot or wearing socks.

Space to exercise
Choose a fairly empty place with room for you to lie full-length. A room with a door you can shut may be quieter and less prone to interruption than a patio or a garden.

Wall
For the wall exercises in Part 5, Level 1, you will need an empty stretch of wall about 1.8 metres (6 feet) wide.

Mat
A tatami mat, which is 1.8 metres (6 feet) long by 0.9 metres (3 feet) wide, and can be rolled up after practice, is ideal for matwork.

Chair
You need a chair without arms that is also the right height for you: when you sit with your behind against the back, you should be able to rest your feet flat on the floor.

Towel
Keep a bath towel handy to roll up and place beneath your knees or feet for floor exercises.

Stick
For the massage, you need a stick about 0.9 metres (3 feet) long and a couple of tennis balls – and a chair close by to place a foot on when massaging calves and thighs.

This book...
Not only does it contain the instructions you need to do the exercises, but it is just the right thickness to rest your head on for the floor exercises in Part 5, Level 3. When exercising lying flat on your back, you need to raise your head slightly to keep it aligned with your spine.

Distractions to avoid...
Listening to music or conversation impedes concentration, so Walkmans, radios and televisions are definitely not part of the equipment you need to practise pilates.

Practice time
Begin by setting aside time three times a week and make a point of sticking to it. Plan for half an hour at first, increasing to an hour after a week or so. Practise at any time of day, but always wait for an hour after eating.

Dreas teaches you to exercise with awareness, so you can effortlessly embody perfect posture. ANDREW FERGUSON, CONSULTANT OSTEOPATH

Joseph Pilates

Joseph Pilates spent more than 30 years studying the body, making himself expert in gymnastics and other physical activities, and researching the effects of exercise on health and fitness. He published his corrective exercises as a self-help fitness method for preventing degenerative illnesses and increasing longevity. He argued passionately in favour of his scientifically researched fitness system, which he claimed to have proven in every detail by experiment and long practice, and which he made freely available to all.

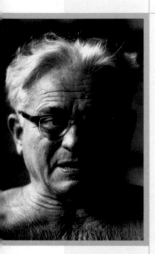

Joseph Pilates, photographed in 1961 at the age of 80. The value of his posture-correcting exercises was recognized among dancers, and his studio had become a focus for professionals in ballet and other performing arts.

Although the pilates exercise system is over half a century old, the name of its founder is missing from most standard reference works. In fact, relatively little is known about his life. The main and almost the only source of information is to be found in *The Pilates Method of Physical and Mental Conditioning*, a book published in 1980 and written by Philip Friedman and Gail Eisen, who studied under a former student of Joseph Pilates. Disseminated by his students and through his own writings, however, his pioneering method of body-conditioning is now winning worldwide recognition.

All biographies of Pilates recount how he was born near the North German city of Düsseldorf in 1880 and grew up a frail child, prone to sickness. The threat of developing tuberculosis is said to have spurred him to work at improving his physical fitness, with such success that at the age of 14 he was posing as a model for anatomical drawings. It is hard to believe that the only known facts about the first 32 years of his life are that he built up his body, and that he practised gymnastics, skiing and diving. He is said to have worked in Britain from 1912 to 1914 as a circus performer, a boxer and a self-defence instructor. During the 1914–18 war, he was interned in England as a German national, and developed his fitness skills by teaching them to fellow internees.

Back in Germany after the war, he is said to have influenced Rudolph von Laban, originator of the widely used system of dance notation. Soon after, in 1923, he emigrated to the USA and settled in New York.

Pilates' New York studio

In a new country Pilates became a pioneer. He set up a studio in New York. In 1934 he published a booklet, *Your Health*, which shows some of the exercise apparatus that has become the hallmark of his system. He gained great respect, and from 1939 he could boast a vast and varied client list, from writers such as Christopher Isherwood to dancers from the New York City Ballet.

Over the years he honed and polished his method, refining it down to the core exercises he published in 1945 in his booklet, *Return to Life Through Contrology*, which he co-wrote with one William John Miller. Photographs illustrated each exercise, and the master himself, now over 60, demonstrated each step for the camera. The exercises in this booklet clearly hang together as a compact and simple system with a clear goal. Through Pilates' writings, and through his students, his system was passed on, after his death in 1967, to the future, to us.

The cult of exercise swept through the USA from the mid-1800s. These illustrations are reproduced from a book, Therapeutics of Activity *by Andrew A. Gour of the Chicago University College of Osteopathy, published in 1923. The exercises are based on Per Henrik Ling's influential Swedish gymnastics system, and many of them closely resemble the exercises taught by Joseph Pilates.*

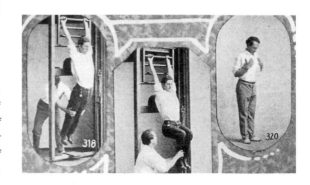

The pioneers

While Joseph Pilates grew up, physical fitness crazes swept through the West. In 1793 Johann Friedrich Guts Muths, a German teacher inspired by the ancient Olympic games, published the first fitness training manual, *Gymnastics for the Young*. It fired a German teacher, Friedrich Ludwig Jahn, to develop exercises for his pupils, aimed at strengthening physique through intensive training on apparatus he designed – the parallel bars and rings. And it inspired a Swedish fencing instructor, Per Henrik Ling, to devise a system of 'medical gymnastics' to strengthen the body through floor movements and his 'Swedish massage'. Both systems spread through Europe and the USA. Jahn's

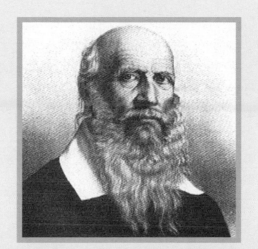

'turning' was the basis of modern Olympic gymnastics, while Ling's more gentle, rhythmic, free-flowing exercises, known as 'Swedish Drill', undoubtedly influenced Joseph Pilates.

Timeline: The concept of physical fitness

This timeline traces the development of fitness training through the 19th century. By 1890 Pilates was studying contemporary fitness training methods intensively, trying to find ways of strengthening his weak body.

- **1800** Denmark introduces physical exercise into the school curriculum.

- **1811** Friedrich Ludwig Jahn, a Prussian secondary school teacher, founds the *Turnverein* ('Turners'), an association of gymnasts, and designs the parallel and horizontal bars, the rings, the balance beam and the pommel horse.

- **1813** The Swedish Gymnastics Institute is founded in Stockholm by Per Henrik Ling, a romantic novelist and fencing master, to teach 'medical gymnastics'.

- **1826** Jahn's revolutionary new gymnastics exercises are taught at Harvard College, USA, by Charles Fallen, a radical German professor.

- **1828** Thomas Arnold, headmaster of Rugby, a British public (fee-paying) school for boys, introduces sports as a method of character-building.

- **1848** The American Turners, the first US gymnastics club, is founded in Cincinnati, Ohio, by German political refugees.

- **1850** Pioneering British educationalist Frances Buss introduces gymnastics at a London school for ladies. She designs loose-fitting gymnastics clothing to replace laced corsets.

- **1857** American educator Catherine Beecher publishes *Physiology and Calisthenics for Schools and Families* to promote calisthenics. This ancient

rhythmic exercise system has been recommended for women by Per Henrik Ling to improve their health.

- **1860** Amherst College, at the University of Massachusetts, USA, establishes the first chair of physical education.

- **1880** Joseph Hubertus Pilates is born in Düsseldorf in the newly unified state of Germany.

- **1893** Swami Vivekenanda, a yogi from India, tours the USA to promote knowledge of yoga.

- **1896** Men's gymnastic events are included in the revived Olympic Games, held in Athens.

The growth of Pilates

Joseph Pilates was born into a world buzzing with excitement over discovery after astonishing discovery about how the body works. 'What has been accomplished within the past ten years as regards knowledge of the causes, prevention, and treatment of disease transcends what would have been regarded a quarter of a century ago as the wildest and most impossible speculation', wrote Austin Flint, the American physiologist who, three years before Pilates' birth, recorded the effects of posture and exercise on the pulse. Pilates developed his fitness method in tandem with the spread of interest in exercise and in response to new knowledge about the health of the human body and the mind.

Around the turn of the 19th century, when Pilates was working out his ideas, the focus of medical research was turning from a search for cures for infectious diseases to investigating chronic and degenerative diseases and how the body maintains health. The stethoscope was invented in 1819 by a French physician, Réné Laennec, and in 1830 the principle of the microscope was discovered by Joseph Lister, a London wine merchant. Using these devices, physicians could listen to the body and look closely at its tissues. Ideas spread internationally even then. The French chemist Louis Pasteur experimented with a microscope and discovered the existence of germs; and three years later Lister, by then a surgeon, inaugurated the era of antiseptic surgery when he sprayed his operating theatre with carbolic acid to kill germs. The century ended with Roentgen's discovery of x-rays, which allowed physicians to see inside the body.

Understanding how energy is produced from diet was a 19th-century achievement. An American writer, Sylvester Graham, studied eating habits and concluded that good diet is essential to health. He published his recommendations in 1839: eat vegetables, fruit, and wholewheat bread; avoid fried meat, alcohol, and refined wheat flour; and eat slowly. A year later, a Swiss chemist discovered that calcium is important for healthy bones, and by the 1870s vegetarian diet was being championed by an American surgeon, John Harvey Kellogg, who made grain-based breakfast cereals. Eventually, in 1895, an agricultural chemist working in the US Department of Agriculture measured the energy produced by eating different foods by applying the kilocalorie to food, and the science of dieting was born.

The essential ingredient: balance

Pilates contributed vigorously to the debate on health issues, railing in print against heart disease – the result of poor diet. He denounced the flat feet and curved spines he saw around him, the postural defects caused by poorly designed furniture, and the unbalanced exercises of other physical culture trainers, which distorted the body. Twentieth-century advances in sports physiology have proved Pilates right: we understand the defects, as well as the benefits, of fitness crazes.

Most exercise systems and sports lack a key ingredient: balance. While weight training, for instance, maximizes muscular strength, and aerobics increases stamina, pilates exercises focus on balancing the actions of the body's whole structure: the skeleton, the joints and muscles, and the major organs. They promote flexibility as well as strength and stamina, and they integrate the different actions of joints and muscles into coordinated, efficient movements. This is structural fitness.

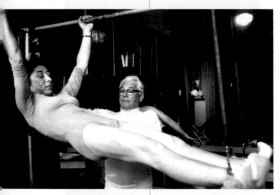

Joseph Pilates supervises a client in his gymnasium on 8th Avenue in New York City on equipment he designed himself. In August 1925, Pilates patented a design for his Universal Reformer, a bed fitted with springs that could be used for resistance when toning the body. The idea is said to have occurred to him while he was working with sick internees during World War I in Britain.

Timeline: The fitness route to health

During the 20th century understanding the role of hygiene, diet, sunlight and fresh air in preventing illness led to a new concept of personal responsibility for maintaining health, and renewed confidence in health-giving exercises for men and women. This timeline shows how pilates developed in response to better knowledge of physiology and of the health effects of exercise.

- **1880** Birth of Joseph Pilates.

- **1893** A test to measure metabolism (the body's production of energy) is devised by German physiologist Adolf Magnus-Levy.

- **1894** X-rays are discovered by a German physicist, Wilhelm Roentgen.

- **1895** Energy produced by eating different foods is successfully measured using the kilocalorie.

- **1903** The electrocardiograph for measuring the heart rate is pioneered by Dutch physiologist Willem Einthoven.

- **1910** The exchange of oxygen and carbon dioxide between the lungs and the blood is discovered by August Krogh and Johannes Lindhard at Copenhagen University.

- **1912** A heart attack is diagnosed in a living person by an American physician, James B. Herrick. It may be due to a blood clot and need not be fatal.

- **1912** Vitamin B is isolated in Japan and vitamin A in the U.S.

- **1912** Joseph Pilates arrives in Britain, where he works as a circus performer and gymnast.

- **1913** Hardening of the arteries (called atherosclerosis) is caused by excess cholesterol and animal fats in the diet, reports Nikolai Anichkov, a pioneering Russian pathologist.

- **1914–18** Joseph Pilates is interned during the Great War.

- **1919–20** Joseph Pilates returns to Germany, where he works as a fitness trainer to the Hamburg police force.

- **1920** Danish scientist August Krogh wins the Nobel Prize for medicine for discovering the role of the capillaries in blood flow around the body.

- **1921** Heart disease overtakes tuberculosis as the major cause of death in the U.S.

- **1923** Joseph Pilates emigrates to the USA. He marries, settles in New York and opens a studio.

- **1923** Discovery of the role of sunlight in producing vitamin D sets off a fashion for beach holidays and outdoor sports and leisure pursuits.

- **1925** Joseph Pilates patents his Universal Reformer, a device for toning the muscles, based on springs.

- **1927** The Harvard Fatigue Laboratory opens at Harvard University, USA, and initiates new research into the effects of exercise on the body.

- **1929** High blood pressure is linked to heart disease by Samuel Albert Levine at Harvard Medical School, USA.

- **1933** Cancer-causing chemicals, called carcinogens, are found in polluted air, auto exhausts, and cigarette smoke.

- **1934** Joseph Pilates publishes *Your Health*, a booklet in which he sets out his ideas on maintaining personal health and fitness.

- **1945** Joseph Pilates publishes his exercises in his second booklet, *Return to Life Through Contrology*.

- **1954** Two American epidemiologists present dramatic evidence that smoking is linked with lung cancer and coronary heart disease.

- **1967** The first scientific conference on exercise physiology is held at the American College of Sports Medicine, USA, and attended by pioneers of physical fitness and exercise physiology.

- **1967** Death of Joseph Pilates.

Mind, brain and body

The association between physical and mental wellbeing was the guiding principle of Joseph Pilates' method, and modern pilates still aims at the coordination of body and mind through exercise. Pilates' thinking will have been influenced by the emergence of the science of psychology. Its birth was marked by Herbert Spencer's *Principles of Psychology*, published in 1855, but this new discipline passed through a controversial adolescence during Pilates' lifetime.

Discoveries of how brain and nerves interact took place in 1811 when a Scottish anatomist, Charles Bell, found that some nerves carry sensation to the brain, while others carry movement instructions. Charles Scott Sherrington, winner of the Nobel Prize for Physiology in 1932, made spectacular discoveries about how the nervous system works.

The emergence of hypnosis and faith-healing may have contributed to Pilates' belief in the healing powers of the mind. Hypnosis, investigated in the 1700s by an Austrian doctor, Franz Mesmer, was revived in the 1800s by James Braid, a Scottish surgeon; and faith healing was publicized in the late 1800s by a French neurophysiologist, Jean Martin Charcot, and by Mary Baker Eddy, the New England founder of the Christian Science movement

The flowering of pilates took place after the death of Joseph Pilates in 1967 and coincided with the emergence of neuropsychology – the study of the brain and its connection with the nervous system. This was made possible by introduction of brain-imaging devices such as CAT, PET and MRI scans. Just as the microscope and the x-ray during the 19th and early 20th century enabled physiologists to see inside the body, these devices have enabled them to probe the brain – to map, for example, the areas responsible for movement in the different parts of the body (see pages 36–37). From this research is rapidly emerging a new understanding of the effects of movement and exercise on body and the mind, the interaction between the left and right sides of the brain and the body, and the development of primitive reflexes, which have a profound effect on the way we learn to stand and move.

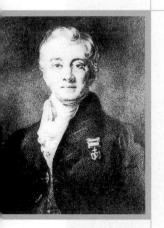

Scottish anatomist Charles Bell, whose Nervous System of the Human Body, *published in 1830, was a beacon in the understanding of how the brain controls movement.*

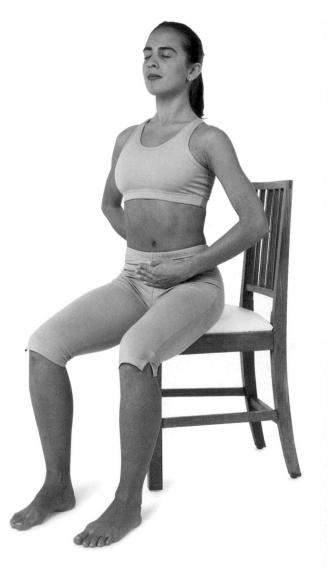

Timeline: Fitness and the mind

This timeline traces landmarks in the advancement of knowledge about psychology, the physiology of the nervous system, and the power of the mind in healing during Joseph Pilates' lifetime, and it covers the period of rapid spread of his exercise system following his death.

■ **1877** The first laboratory for experimental psychology is opened in Leipzig by German psychologist Wilhelm Max Wundt, who emphasizes the use of the scientific method.

■ **1877** Charles Darwin's *Biographical Sketch of an Infant*, the diary of the development of his son, is the first study of child psychology.

■ **1882** Hypnosis is used by Viennese physician Joseph Breuer to treat a girl suffering from hysteria, pioneering the development of psychoanalysis.

■ **1891** Spinal reflexes (e.g., the knee jerk) and the synapses or junctions between nerves are discovered by English neurophysiologist Charles Scott Sherrington.

■ **1899–1900** Sigmund Freud, Viennese neurosurgeon, publishes his ideas in *The Interpretation of Dreams*.

■ **1905** Carl Gustav Jung, a Swiss psychologist, publishes *Psychology of Dementia Praecox*, breaking new ground in the study of mental illness.

■ **1900** The hormone adrenalin is discovered by chemists at Johns Hopkins Medical School, who produce it synthetically as a drug. It is later discovered to be produced by the body in response to stress.

■ **1910** Autosuggestive healing is introduced by French pharmacist Emile Coué, who has studied hypnotism.

■ **1921** The Rorschach test is introduced by Swiss psychiatrist Hermann Rorschach to probe the unconscious.

■ **1925** The Menninger Clinic opens in Kansas, headed by Charles F. Menninger, a physician whose total environment approach revolutionizes treatment of mental illness.

■ **1928** The mechanism by which nerves carry messages to and from the brain is worked out by English physiologist Edgar Douglas Adrian.

■ **1940s–50s** The concept of stress is formulated by Hans Selye, a Canadian physiologist, who notices that patients with different diseases often have similar symptoms.

■ **early 1970s** The CT (computed tomography) scan is developed. It produces cross-sectional images of the brain, giving physiologists a visual image of the inside of the brain.

■ **mid-1970s** The PET (positron emission tomography) scan is introduced, which enables physiologists to measure the metabolism (energy-consumption) of the brain, including changes in oxygen consumption and blood flow, and the production of neurotransmitter chemicals by the brain during exercise.

■ **1975** Peter Blythe establishes the Institute for Neuro-Physiological Psychology in the UK, to study the primitive reflexes of children. Neural therapy for children with learning difficulties is founded by Sally Goddard.

■ **early 1980s** Magnetic resonance imaging (MRI scans) use radio waves to produce detailed images of the brain

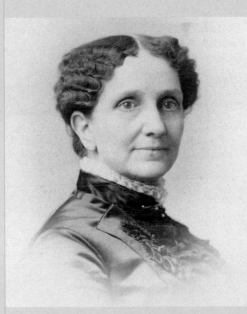

In 1875, Mary Baker, an American divorcée, published Science and Health, *in which she presented her ideas on faith-healing, based on the Bible. In 1879, she established the Church of Christ, Scientist.*

Pilates for the 21st century

Pilates wanted his exercises to be a fitness aid for everyone, but only after his death did they spread beyond the domain of dancers and other performers. In 1973 I opened my studio in London and began exploring ways of adapting them to meet the different requirements of my diverse clients. They include working people keen to keep fit and stay in shape, mothers wanting to regain strength and flexibility after delivery, and dancers anxious to improve their technique. The result is a pilates-based exercise method which, by responding to new scientific discoveries about how the brain and body interact, is taking structural fitness and body balance into the 21st century.

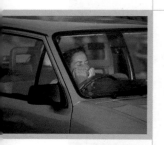

We have total freedom of movement. We can fly, drive, take a train, take a bus. The message is: don't walk.

Pilates' core exercises are still the basis of the matwork in modern pilates, but his method is neither rigid or strictly controlled. Indeed, although he specified that his exercises be performed in the order and according to the instructions he set down, Pilates worked one-to-one with his clients, adapting his method to suit each individual. Some people need to concentrate on relaxing the neck and shoulders, others on loosening the hamstrings. Consequently, between the 1970s and the turn of the 20th century, fitness teachers have taken his method in many different directions.

A major development has been the adaptation of the core exercises carried out against a wall. Level 1, Stage 2 (pages 88–124) has mainly wall exercises, while most of the exercises in Level 3 (pages 172–203) are carried out lying down. It is easier for beginners to exercise standing and using a wall or a chair for stability than lying down.

Pilates exercises are very adaptable, and in different studios they are taught in distinctive ways. In some New York studios, for example, exercising is hard and fast, like aerobics. But most trainers, myself included, encourage their clients to exercise thoughtfully, to a slow, controlled rhythm. Some aerobic exercise is essential to health, however, and I recommend aerobics sessions on the exercise ball and the bouncer (see pages 72–75).

Some teachers take classes, but I prefer to work one-to-one. I do not believe in classes for 24, because in my view pilates exercises are not intended for groups. Instructors who teach Pilates' system need to pay special attention to each client's postural and structural needs.

Structural fitness

The concept of structural fitness is not yet well known, although it is seriously applied in professional, competitive sports training and in sports medicine. One reason is that although Pilates' core exercises can be practised by anyone, the instructions in his books may be difficult to follow without personal help, and some of his exercises may be unsuitable for particular individuals. In Part 5 I break down the movements and explain them so they can be followed easily. I also grade the exercises, so they become progressively more demanding. The result is a set of key exercises for beginners of all ages to follow, which provide the tools for achieving structural fitness.

Like most pilates studios, mine is equipped with apparatus, such as the Trapeze, the Reformer, the Barrel and the Wunda Chair. Studio apparatus is useful for exercising during pregnancy, for example (see pages 214–15), for correcting sports injuries, or to help actors speed up development of a particular body shape for a role (see pages 210–11). Yet Pilates demonstrated his exercises without apparatus. He devised a simple system to help people assess their own postural defects and correct them, realign the body, and stretch and tone muscles using nothing more than floor space.

The next three chapters are a preparation for the exercises. Parts 2 and 3 explain the body systems involved in exercise, and I hope you will return to them time and again, because practising the exercises makes you want to know more about how your body works. And Part 4 helps you assess your body and identify its needs.

Timeline: Fitness in the 20th century

Renewed enthusiasm for fitness arose in the West during the 1970s. Innovative exercise systems such as jogging and aerobics resulted from discoveries in sports science, while interest in the wisdom of the ancient East made yoga and martial arts such as taijiquan (tai-chi ch'uan) popular. As the ill effects of a sedentary lifestyle became widely understood, exercises to restore structural balance, such as Alexander Technique and pilates, gained popularity. At the beginning of the 1990s there were only four pilates studios in London; by 1999, there were at least 20, and pilates organizations had been established in European cities, in Australia and New Zealand, Cape Town, Tokyo, and all over North America. This timeline traces the late-20th century spread of pilates alongside other fitness systems.

■ **1950s** Schools of the Chinese art of tai jiquan (t'ai chi-ch'uan) are opened in Taiwan and the USA by respected Chinese instructors who have fled the Communist revolution in China.

■ **1950s** B.K.S. Iyengar, a leading yoga teacher of the 20th century, tours Europe and the USA giving classes and demonstrations.

■ **1970** The New York Marathon on September 23 has 126 starters, who run four times around Central Park. The Chicago Marathon follows in 1977 and the London Marathon in 1981.

■ **1970** A pilates studio opens at London's Contemporary Dance Company, run by Alan Herdman who has studied pilates in New York.

■ **1970** Nautilus exercise machines, based on resistance equipment to prevent bone loss in astronauts, is marketed in the USA by an engineer, Arthur Young.

■ **1972–73** Pilates studios are set up in Israel for the Bathsheba Company by British pilates teacher Alan Herdman.

■ **1973** The efficacy of the Alexander Technique is publicized by Nikolaas Tinbergen, winner of the Nobel Prize for Medicine, inspiring widespread new interest in the practice.

■ **1973** Andreas Reyneke, a former dancer and a pilates teacher, opens his London studio to teach pilates-based fitness exercises to individuals.

■ **1977** Ida P. Rolf, American physiologist, publishes *Rolfing,* her seminal work on structural integration and body-balancing, based on her study of the connective tissues.

■ **1977** *The Complete Book of Running* by James S. Fixx appears in the USA, heralding a new craze for jogging.

My Body-Conditioning Studio, seen here as it was furnished in the 1970s, was only the second pilates studio to open in London after Joseph Pilates' death in 1967.

■ **1980** The first brief biography of Joseph Pilates is published 100 years after his birth.

■ **1980s** A craze for aerobics training to increase endurance and stamina follows the publication of research into exercise physiology in the USA and the Scandinavian countries.

■ **1986** A pilates studio opens in Sydney, Australia, run by Allan Menendes, an athlete who studied pilates in London.

■ **1998–99** Pilates studios open in Cape Town, South Africa.

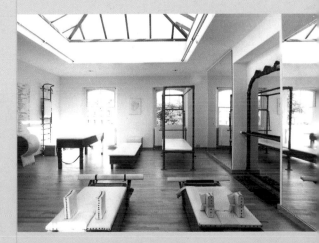

part 2
body structure

Structural fitness is the one
 essential fitness on which
all other fitness depends.

JOHN L. STIRK, OSTEOPATH

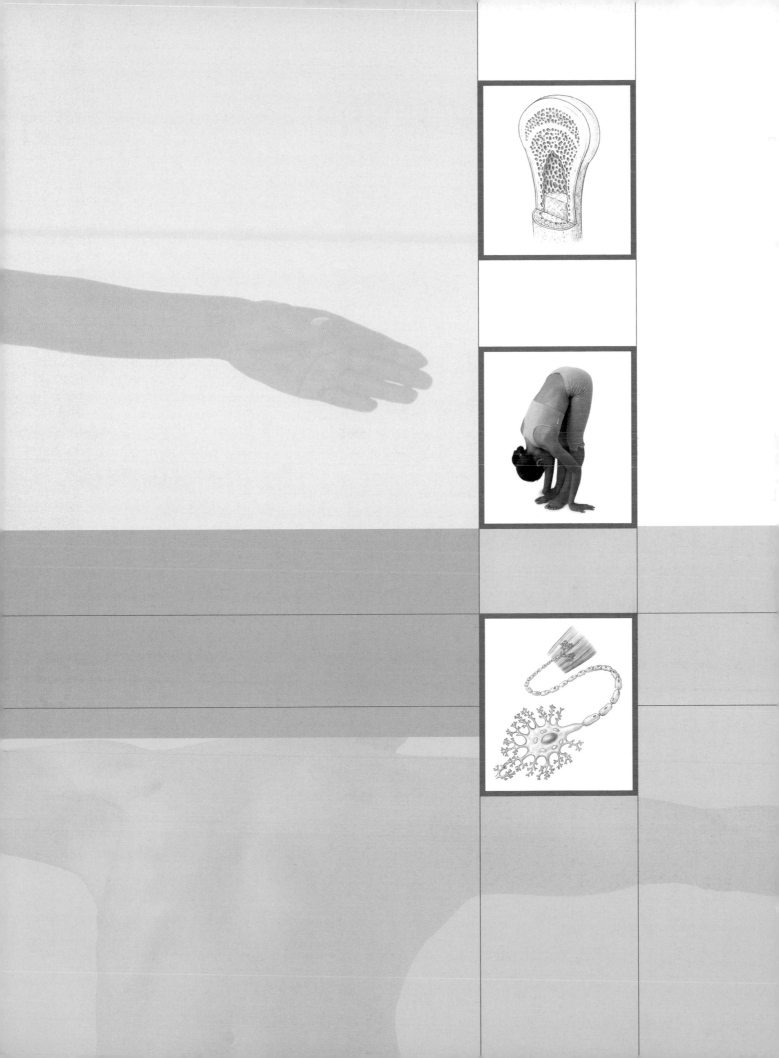

Time machine

The body is a wonder of precision engineering. Its structural frame, the skeleton, is strong and resilient but light and flexible. More than 200 bones work in partnership with the joints and muscles to stabilize the body and move it. The brain governs their actions, transmitting electrochemical impulses along the nerves to stimulate muscles to contract. From birth, children naturally explore the body's full range of movement, but stressful yet inactive 21st-century lifestyles mean that adults must exercise to keep fit. Time ensures that like all mechanical structures, gravity, movement and injuries compress, stress and wear the body. A holistic approach to exercise is the way to repair damage and restore and maintain structural fitness.

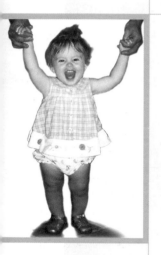

Babies in the first months of life find it exciting just to discover the postural reflexes and explore the balance mechanism.

The body is a time machine. From the moment of conception to the day of death it works steadily through a development programme written in its genes. The body is a self-maintaining system, and left to develop without hindrance, it is capable of attaining and maintaining its natural levels of strength and fitness throughout its lifespan. But modern living tends to hinder the body's efforts to maintain structural fitness. A sedentary lifestyle eventually inhibits movement, and the effects can be devastating. 'Use it or lose it' is a warning commonly given to the elderly, which applies equally to the young.

It is now thought that normal structural development may be threatened by factors that affect the unborn child. Drugs such as alcohol and nicotine taken in small quantities during pregnancy are known to inhibit the developing responses of the fetus. Medical researchers believe that the swimming movements babies make during birthing may stimulate reflexes that enable them to develop coordinated movement (see pages 38–39). A cesarean birth may prevent the emergence of these reflexes and inhibit an infant from developing balanced movement. In the first year, baby bouncers and bulky nappies may affect the natural alignment of hips and legs, with an adverse effect on posture and movement.

Standing tall

The body has to operate under the weight of gravity and is subject to physical tensions and stresses. Over millennia it has evolved a structure that enables it to deal efficiently with these forces. Its various parts are aligned to form a columnar shape that transmits weight efficiently from the skull to the pelvis to the feet. The joints where its component parts meet—the neck, the shoulders, the vertebrae, the hips, the knees, and the ankles—are flexible so that the columnar structure can be maintained when the body is moving.

Poor posture destroys this symmetry with disastrous results. A body with drooping head, rounded shoulders, and protruding pelvis has to work hard to maintain core stability against gravity and changing ground levels when walking. Body structures and systems are interconnected and interactive, so any one of these structural faults throws the rest of the body out of alignment causing fatigue, pain and, in time, permanent damage.

Injuries to the body, especially to the joints, affect balance and overall mechanical efficiency. As they heal, function returns, but the balance of the body may have been affected. It quickly compensates for even minor injuries: a blister on a heel changes the way you walk, so a serious injury can affect stance or gait permanently.

Many other factors, from emotional lows to the way you lift heavy objects, can cause structural imbalances. The older you are, the more damage you are likely to have accumulated and the less likely you are to be aware of it. To help you understand how structural fitness exercises can correct disturbances in your body's natural balance, this chapter explains body structure and and shows how neglect and injury can affect it.

Time and habit

'Behaviour bears witness to a given structure,' wrote Ida Rolf, the American physiologist who explored body alignment and posture. If you spend most of your life sitting and slumping, and do not correct your posture, you will become increasingly disabled as you get older. Structural fitness exercises can correct postural defects and enable you to remain flexible and mobile into old age.

The effects of time

Develop the habit of standing tall and you will still be standing tall in your later years. But let your shoulders droop, and:

- Habitually rounded shoulders will eventually cause your chest to cave in, lengthening and weakening the extensor muscles at the back of your chest.
- As a result, the muscle that helps hold your shoulder blades flat against your ribs will weaken and fail to balance the action of the rhomboid muscles, which act in opposition, pulling your shoulder blades up.
- To counterbalance your shoulders, your head will begin to tilt back. Its weight will fall on your throat and on the prevertebral muscles (see page 48) at the back of your neck.
- Your chin will begin to poke forward, leading your head, and your eye sockets will tilt upwards.
- The muscles of your upper chest and back are consequently all thrown out of balance so that your shoulder joint gradually rotates forwards.
- The palms of your hands will gradually turn to face backwards. In time this will restrict the range of movement of your arm joints.

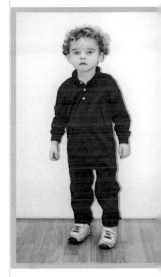

Like most young children, this three-year-old has naturally good posture. Even a toddler who has just learned to walk instinctively remains upright while moving its insecurely balanced body weight and spontaneously adjusting to the unexpected.

If slumping and slouching become habitual and their effects on the body are not corrected by exercise, the forward-leaning posture becomes ingrained. The muscles of the upper back become permanently stretched, the underused muscles of the chest weaken, the spine bows, and the shoulders collapse forwards. Eventually it may be possible to walk only with a stick.

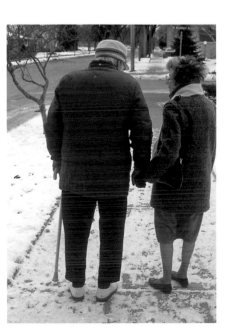

Form and function

The main structures of the body begin to form when we are still just a fertilized egg. The spine starts to develop three weeks after conception; by the fifth week, limbs appear; and by the eighth week the fetus has a soft skeleton of cartilage, which is hardening into bone. A newborn baby quickly begins to explore its ability to move and to adjust the relationship between different body parts for balance and stability. Through childhood the body develops the full vocabulary of movement, but after maturity much of this movement potential is lost through disuse. Inactivity causes bones to lose calcium and become brittle, half-used joints to lose flexibility, and muscles to weaken.

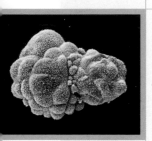

Three weeks after conception, the fertilized egg is a fluid-filled sphere. Cells in its outer shell are already transforming rapidly into cartilage, connective tissue, bone, muscle, and blood cells.

Your skeleton is your framework. It gives your body its human shape and determines the space it occupies, its height, width, and breadth. It shapes the spaces occupied by the major organs, from brain to bladder. The skeleton can be strengthened and the balance of its separate parts altered, but its measurements are fixed at maturity.

From the skull to the metatarsals in the toes, our bones were formed before we were born. They developed from cartilage, a soft, bendable tissue made of the proteins elastin and collagen. From the seventh week after conception, the tough, twisted collagen fibres are gradually impregnated with calcium and phosphorus, which make bone tissue hard and resistant but pliable so that it does not break easily. All through childhood and adolescence the bones lengthen by this same process.

Kids and exercise

Children need to run and play naturally so they develop an instinct for good carriage and natural movement. Rigid posture and rigorous exercise training can inhibit this natural body sense. A child's body changes fast, and during adolescence bone growth accelerates. The spine grows fastest in girls between 9 and 14 years, and in boys between 12 and 17 years. The growth spurt begins in the lumbar spine – the low back – before puberty, then the thoracic spine or upper back catches up, and the sacral or pelvic skeleton matures last. During these years it is good to spend time playing active games and learning sports. Teenagers need plenty of rest and sleep, but they need exercise because prolonged sitting encourages slumping. This compresses the lungs, stomach, and other organs of the chest and abdomen, restricting breathing and affecting mood.

However, sports trainers working with young people must keep the growth spurt in mind. The cartilage of the hip is soft in adolescents and may be damaged by forcefully bending the knee up to the waist. The rapidly growing bones are fragile and easily stress-fractured; the muscles develop more slowly and can become taut, making the limbs hard to control. The tibia, or main leg bone, may lengthen more rapidly than the calf muscles, so that a teenager may be temporarily unable to place the heel fully on the ground and may start walking on tiptoe. Adolescents need a diet high in calcium, phosphorus and other minerals, and vitamins C and D.

Stability and mobility

Babies begin life with some 350 soft bones, but as they grow, and the cartilage ossifies or hardens, many bones fuse. The adult skeleton has only about 206, with cartilage in specialized areas, such as the ends of bones where they meet and form joints. Pairs and groups of bones are bound together tightly by ropelike ligaments of strong fibrous tissue. The skeleton works as a unit, a movement in one part causing adjustments elsewhere. The body is rarely still, and the joints are where stability and mobility meet. Joints maintain stability at fixed locations, such as the knees and hips, while allowing the bones to move in response to the pull of muscles. To make this possible, many different joints are needed at key points in the body.

The spine

Your spine is your body's central axis. It supports your head and transmits the weight of your whole upper body down to your pelvis. Its 33 bones or vertebrae interlock and are bound firmly together by ligaments, yet each pair is cushioned by a cartilage layer and separated by a cartilage disk, which allows a small degree of movement. The spine becomes s-shaped as a baby learns to walk. Its curves enable it to withstand the stresses imposed by moving and rotating in different directions:

- The atlas and axis are the two strong vertebrae at the top of the spine that support the skull. They form a joint that allows it to nod and turn.
- The ribs are attached to the upper back or thoracic vertebrae.
- All the weight of the upper body is channelled down to the fifth lumbar vertebra, which forms a slightly movable joint with the sacrum and the pelvis. The weight travels from the sacrum, around the pelvis to the hips and thighs.
- The sacrum is the strong shield-shaped bone at the base of the spine, which forms the back of the pelvis.
- The coccyx provides attachment for the structures of the pelvic floor and moves very slightly when the pelvic floor is lifted.

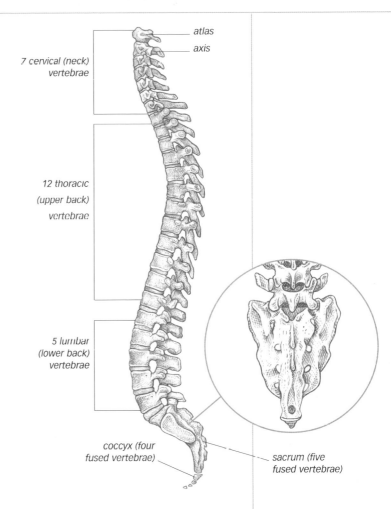

atlas
axis

7 cervical (neck) vertebrae

12 thoracic (upper back) vertebrae

5 lumbar (lower back) vertebrae

coccyx (four fused vertebrae)

sacrum (five fused vertebrae)

Joints of the spine

Thick cartilage disks cushion the vertebrae against gravitational compression and injury. They compress to let the spine bend forwards, sideways, and backwards, and to rotate. Jarring the spine may damage the disk, and you may feel intense pain if, in time, its pulpy centre is squeezed out and irritates a major nerve. Gliding joints allow the spines of neighbouring vertebrae to pass smoothly over each other.

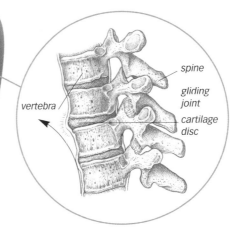

spine

gliding joint

cartilage disc

vertebra

Many pairs of muscles are attached to the vertebrae to bend and flex the spine. Although cartilage disks and gliding joints allow each pair of vertebrae only a small degree of movement, all those tiny movements add up to such marvellous flexibility that you can almost bend yourself in half.

29

The connective tissues

Bones, cartilage and the ligaments that bind the bones together are all connective tissues. So are the muscles and the tissues that encase organs such as the lungs and the stomach, and hold them in place. Blood, which is manufactured by cells in the bones, is a type of connective tissue. All begin to develop in the first weeks of life, before the fertilized egg has become an embryo.

Bones, muscles and blood all have a specialized role, yet they also have a collective function: to support and cushion the vital organs. By binding and separating muscles, connective tissue shapes much of the body surface. Its work is visible in the tightly packed muscle layers beneath the skin on an athlete's lean body, and in the developed muscle structure of the body-builder.

Interconnecting system

The connective tissues form an interconnecting network all over the body, so strain and flaccidity in one area is rapidly communicated body-wide. Loss of elasticity in the connective tissues is immediately evident in collapse of posture. The organs inside the lower abdomen are held up by the pelvic floor, the hammock of thin muscle sheets and membranes of connective tissue slung horizontally across the base of the pelvic girdle. When this complex structure loses tone, it sags, pulling the pelvis and lower spine out of alignment. Standing and walking become hard work because the pelvis is thrown out of alignment, and pressure on the lumbar spine causes low back pain.

The dividing lines between the different types of connective tissue are often indistinct. The skeletal muscles, themselves a form of connective tissue, are wrapped in a sheet of fascia, a transparent but tough covering that holds the muscle fibres in alignment. At each end of the muscle, the fascia forms tendons – the strong, fibrous cords that fix the muscles to bones. Muscle efficiency depends to a high degree on the elasticity and responsiveness of the connective tissue. Loss of tone adversely affects movement, and also mood, no doubt, for its health and strength are essential to the body's sense of internal wellbeing.

What makes muscle different from other forms of connective tissue is its ability to contract. The muscle tissue of the heart makes its continuous, rhythmic contractions independently, without stimulation from the brain. The smooth muscle lining the blood vessels and intestines contracts slowly, forming wavelike movements that propel nutrients and blood along. And skeletal or voluntary muscles contract rapidly when stimulated by an electrochemical impulse from the brain carried by the nerves that supply them. This is the mechanism that enables muscles to act on joints and so move bones.

The long bones

Bone is a type of connective tissue. It has a hard outer shell and softer tissue inside, served by nerves, arteries, veins and lymph vessels. Bones are light because they have a strong central honeycomb structure filled with bone marrow, from which blood cells are made.

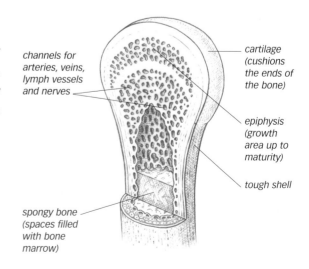

channels for arteries, veins, lymph vessels and nerves

cartilage (cushions the ends of the bone)

epiphysis (growth area up to maturity)

tough shell

spongy bone (spaces filled with bone marrow)

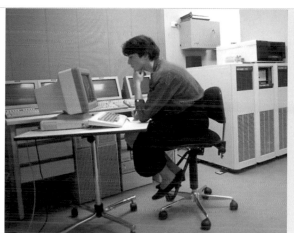

Sitting and standing

Slouched sitting, or standing with the weight on one hip can destroy the angle at which the pelvis naturally tilts. The muscles that raise the body from sitting to standing shorten with too much sitting, and if slouching becomes an ingrained habit the effect on posture is disastrous:

- The abdominal muscles weaken and the stomach protrudes.
- Strain on the lower back causes the curve in the lumbar spine to deepen and its supporting muscles to shorten. This can be painful.
- The pelvis, forced out of its natural alignment, tilts forward.
- The unnatural angle of the hips causes pain in the lower back.

Connective tissue types—the pelvis

The pelvic floor

The basin-shaped pelvis cradles the abdominal organs. The pelvic floor is a strip of muscle and connective tissue slung across the pelvis from the coccyx (tailbone) to the pubic symphysis in front, supporting the organs. If it weakens and sags the abdomen protrudes; and the muscles of the bladder and rectum, and the vagina in women, become stressed and lose tone.

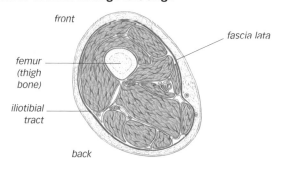

pubic symphysis

pelvic floor

coccyx

rectum

The pelvic tilt

When the pelvic girdle is correctly positioned, the opening at its base is not parallel with the floor. It is designed to transmit the weight of the upper body to the hip joints, and for this it needs to be inclined forward at an angle of about 60°. The correct tilt brings the the joint at the front, called the pubic symphysis, roughly level with the base of the coccyx.

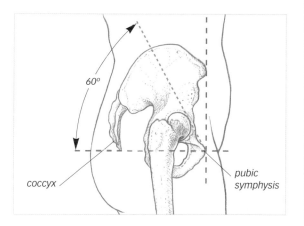

60°

coccyx

pubic symphysis

The muscle sheath

The fascia lata is a layer of connective tissue that fits like a stocking around the thigh, holding the internal structures in place. It is tough enough to take the stress of the tensor fasciae latae muscle (see page 56), which inserts into it and tightens a thick band of connective tissue called the iliotibial tract. This runs down the side of the thigh and braces the knee, especially when you stand on one foot.

Cross-section through left thigh

front

fascia lata

femur (thigh bone)

iliotibial tract

back

Head to toe

The skull may feel solid, but like the rest of the skeleton it consists of many bones separated by joints, although they do not move. There are joints between the sacrum and the pelvic girdle, which loosen and widen a little during pregnancy. And some joints, notably those between pairs of vertebrae or spinal bones, have limited movement (see page 29). All these joints are exceptions, however, because most of the joints of the trunk and limbs are freely movable. These are at the junctions of long bones, and they let you fold your limbs in, or flex them, and stretch them out, or extend them. Their movements are balanced by the actions of muscles, which maintain equal tension on either side of each joint. The result is to stabilize the body structure to allow dynamic posture and active movement.

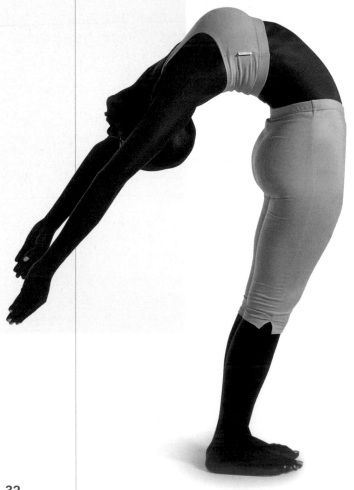

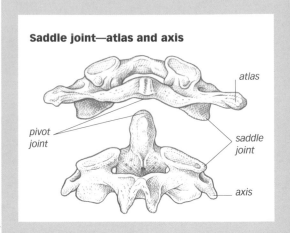

Saddle joint—atlas and axis

atlas

pivot joint

saddle joint

axis

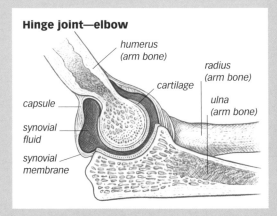

Hinge joint—elbow

humerus (arm bone)

radius (arm bone)

cartilage

capsule

ulna (arm bone)

synovial fluid

synovial membrane

Atlas and axis

The skull rests on depressions in the atlas, the top cervical vertebra, forming a saddle joint that allows it to rock up and down, as in nodding.

The second cervical vertebra has a bony knob, which protrudes into a hole in the atlas to form a pivot joint. This turns the head left and right.

The elbow

Like the knee and the finger and toe joints, the elbow is a hinge joint: it flexes or bends in one direction. But the tendons of many muscles are attached to the bones to enable the forearm to rotate at the elbow, as well as to lift and lower, so it is one of the more mobile joints. Freely movable joints like those of the limbs are called synovial joints because they are sealed inside a capsule of fibrous tissue, and the cavity between the bones is filled with lubricating fluid secreted by the surrounding synovial membrane. Cartilage protects the bones from friction.

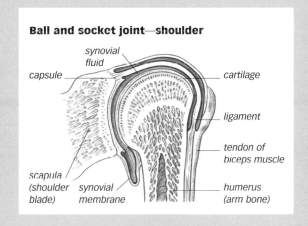

Ball and socket joint—shoulder

- capsule
- synovial fluid
- cartilage
- ligament
- tendon of biceps muscle
- scapula (shoulder blade)
- synovial membrane
- humerus (arm bone)

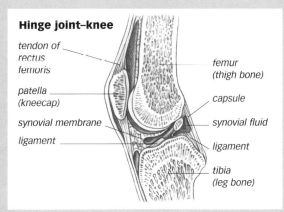

Hinge joint–knee

- tendon of rectus femoris
- patella (kneecap)
- synovial membrane
- ligament
- femur (thigh bone)
- capsule
- synovial fluid
- ligament
- tibia (leg bone)

The shoulder

The shoulder and the hip are the most flexible joints – the shoulder joint can turn through almost 360°. They are called ball and socket joints because a ball-shaped projection on the humerus (arm bone) and on the femur (thigh bone) fits into a socket on the shoulder and in the hip bone respectively. Five rotator muscles form a cuff around the shoulder joint, which allows the arm to move up, down, forwards, backwards, and to either side, and to rotate in several planes.

The knee

This joint has to bear the weight of the whole body, plus increased pressure during running and jumping. The knee is a hinge joint, but it is the largest and most complex freely movable joint. It can bend, straighten, and rotate a little when bent. A complex of strong ligaments holds the bones in place. The tendon of the rectus femoris muscle is firmly attached to the patella or kneecap, which moves as the knee is flexed and straightened to keep the tendon properly aligned (see page 123).

The feet

The feet take the strain of every weight-bearing movement. The weight of the standing body travels from the body's centre of gravity in the pelvic girdle down the femur or thigh bone and the tibia, the main bone of the leg, to the ankle, where it divides to follow two pathways to the ground. Good posture distributes the weight equally to the heels and forefeet of both feet.

The foot bones form three arches. These transmit the body weight to the ground: the medial arch runs from the calcaneus or heel bone along the first three metatarsals to the great toe; the lateral arch runs parallel to it along the fourth and fifth metatarsals; and the transverse arch spans the cuneiform bones that form the crown of the longitudinal arches. Their wedge shape directs the weight to the forefoot. The foot muscles and their tendons, and

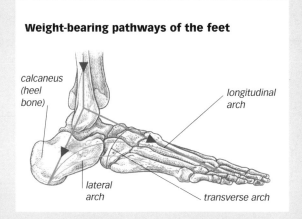

Weight-bearing pathways of the feet

- calcaneus (heel bone)
- longitudinal arch
- lateral arch
- transverse arch

a whole complex of ligaments support the three arches and hold them in alignment. If they are overstretched or weakened, the arches collapse, resulting in flat feet. This reduces the efficiency of the foot in walking and running.

Body and mind

In the early days of brain research, scientists expected to identify a key area of the brain, or a cluster of cells whose function is to make decisions and initiate action. Instead, they found that movement involves cooperation between the body and extensive areas of the brain, from the nerves that fire muscles into action to the parts of the brain where conscious thought is located. Twenty-first-century research proves that 100 years ago, Joseph Pilates was right to emphasize the role of the mind in exercising the body.

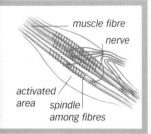

Spindle cells deep in skeletal muscle fibres monitor the stretching of surrounding fibres

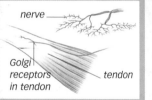

Golgi tendon organs alert the brain to relax muscles when their tendons are subjected to excessive stretching.

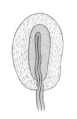

Pacinian corpuscles work with Golgi tendon organs. They fire when a movement begins and when it ends.

All your body systems are interconnected. There is constant interaction between your bones, muscles, and connective tissue network, and that is why letting your foot muscles weaken, for example, can displace your pelvis and cause sciatica, low back pain and tension in your neck and shoulders. But the nervous system is the most extensive of the body's interactive systems. It keeps all structures and systems alert and active even when you are still, asleep or unconscious.

The internal eye

Nerves relay information from your brain to all tissues and organs, and they feed back data from sensors almost everywhere in the body. Sensitive skin surfaces such as the fingertips are especially well supplied with nerves that respond to touch and pain.

Nerves that activate skeletal muscles, tendons, and joints have sensation receptors at the ends. These feed back to the central nervous system (the brain and spinal cord) information about stretch, tension and pressure. They are called proprioceptors ('proprio' means 'oneself') because they update the brain on the location of all body parts, giving it an accurate picture of the positions of your hands, fingers, feet, elbows, head, and so on in relation to each other. And like an air traffic controller's screen, they keep your brain posted on whether limbs are moving, in what direction, and how fast. This information prevents damage. Spindle-shaped cells located among muscle fibres are proprioceptors that make your head jerk up if you nod off when sitting upright. They monitor adjacent fibres, and if their length and tension approach danger point, the spindle cells alert the brain, which signals the muscle to contract. Similarly, Golgi tendon organs respond when muscle tendons are stretched excessively, by alerting the brain to relax the straining muscles. They cause the losing combatant in an arm-wrestling bout to release rather than continue pushing until the tendon tears or the arm breaks. Pacinian corpuscles live in nerve fibres at the junctions between muscles and their tendons, close to Golgi tendon organs. When a muscle moves, its Golgi tendon organs are compressed. They fire once to warn the central nervous system that movement has begun; and when it stops, they fire again.

Automatic movements

Signals from proprioceptors travel along nerves (called 'neurones') to the spinal cord and are relayed to the brain's information processing centres. There they are integrated with data from all over your body, and acted upon. This relaying process begins in the brain stem, the oldest brain area and the seat of unconscious movement. Neurones connect it with the higher brain and with the cerebellum or "small brain" behind it (see pages 34–35).

The cerebellum works at an automatic level to ensure that you move normally without having to think about each movement – imagine always having to concentrate on putting one foot in front of the other. It receives information about body position and movement and, in communication with the higher brain centres, it fine-tunes complex movements, keeping the body balanced and maintaining posture by always keeping one-third of muscle fibres contracted. Persistent clumsiness can signal malfunction because smooth coordination of movements is a major function of this brain area.

Interactive systems

Making movements such as walking and exercising involves the whole mind and body. Data from receptors in muscles, tendons, joints and skin, and from eyes, ears and nose are linked in the brain with input from memory and from brain areas involved in abstract thinking. For example, the brain compares past movement experiences with the current situation, and predicted speeds with actual progress, and makes adjustments. Backup routes are worked out before movement begins, in case of unexpected obstruction. Progress is monitored, and when movement needs to end, inhibition routines are activated to halt moving joints and bones.

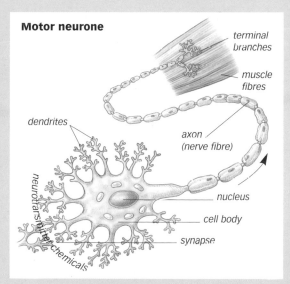

Motor neurone

terminal branches

muscle fibres

dendrites

axon (nerve fibre)

neurotransmitter chemicals

nucleus

cell body

synapse

Nerves link body and mind. They originate in the brain stem; bundles of their long fibres, called axons, form the spinal cord and branch again and again, eventually to connect with the proprioceptors in the body tissues. Nerves that control movement, called motor neurones, transmit electrochemical signals from the brain to the skeletal muscles to initiate or halt movement. Signals from sensors and proprioceptors in the skin, muscles and other tissues travel along sensory nerves to be processed by the brain. Nerves also transmit signals to neighbouring nerves across junctions called synapses via chemicals that transmit electrochemical impulses.

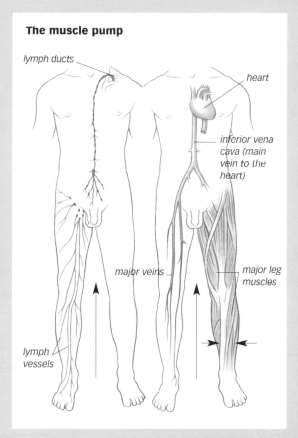

The muscle pump

lymph ducts

heart

inferior vena cava (main vein to the heart)

major veins

major leg muscles

lymph vessels

When you exercise your leg muscles contract and relax, pushing against adjacent veins and lymph vessels. The veins are carrying blood from the feet up to the heart, and the lymph vessels are carrying fluid drained from the tissues to the upper chest, where it returns through ducts into the blood. Both blood and lymph have to flow up the legs and the abdomen to the chest. The muscles contract rhythmically against the vessels, pumping the blood and lymph upwards against gravity.

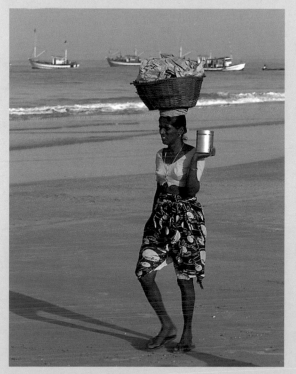

Your body is always moving, so the position of your head is always critical. Aligning it correctly ensures that you can make the most of all the information that your eyes, the organs of hearing and balance in your ears, and the proprioceptors or sensors in your skin and other tissues are transmitting to your brain about the orientation of your body in space.

The exercise experience

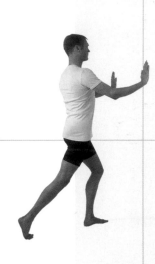

The repetitive movements involved in exercising may engage the higher brain activities only at the learning stage. Once an exercise has been practised enough to be remembered, executing it becomes semi-automatic, like writing. The involvement of the decision-making centres diminishes, and signals affecting the repeated movements are processed by the lower brain.

The brain stem and spinal cord were the earliest parts of the brain to evolve. They begin to form early, in the fifth week of pregnancy, along with message-relaying stations in the midbrain, the hypothalamus (where the nervous and hormone systems interact), and the senses. By week 20 the fetus is making simple movements such as flexion (bending joints) and kicking. Soon, the developing baby can rotate the spine and move the limbs, to suck a thumb, for instance. By the 32nd week the inner ear structures have developed, so the fetus has a sense of orientation and balance and can turn in the womb.

If you have neglected your body for an all-too-sedentary lifestyle, take heart. The lower centres of your brain have never forgotten the movements you used to make with scarcely a conscious thought. Exercise patterns once practised to perfection, then neglected, just need to be practised again to restore their efficiency.

The seat of conscious movement

The upper and largest part of the brain is the cerebrum. Its folds (called "gyri") and fissures (called "sulci") divide it into four lobes. A thin layer of grey matter (nervous tissue containing nerve nuclei) covers it. This is the cerebral cortex, the most evolved part of the brain where conscious thought and decision-making happen. Neurones that activate movement are found in the frontal lobe. Researchers have mapped this area and identified where neurones associated with different parts of the body are located. The brain map on the right shows where some movement areas are sited.

If you are in the later decades of life, be confident that your higher brain centres will always respond to your body's intention to learn new movements. Your neurones, proprioceptors, muscles and tendons will never be too old to learn new movements and exercises. Researchers at Harvard University in the USA have published reports on strength training for people aged over 80, which increased bone strength and density, improved metabolic rate, strengthened muscles (making it easier to climb stairs), increased stability, reduced blood pressure – and, because body and mind work together, gave participants greater optimism about life and living.

The lower brain centres

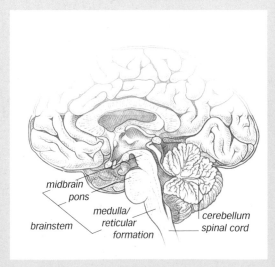

midbrain
pons
brainstem
medulla/
reticular
formation
cerebellum
spinal cord

Cerebellum *Coordinates movement; receives data from proprioceptors, and regulates muscle tone to maintain posture; receives information about orientation from organs of balance.*

Brainstem *Oldest part of the brain, consists of:*
- *Midbrain: organizes and dispatches impulses from motor nerves entering and leaving the brain. Relays visual and auditory information.*
- *Pons: relays data from spinal cord to cerebellum and cerebral cortex.*
- *Medulla: spinal cord interfaces with the brain. Control of vital functions.*
- *Reticular formation: netlike neurone cluster, integrates data from movement receptors in the body, including from muscles that balance the body against gravity. Acting on feedback from decision-making centres, it may increase information flow to and from these muscles, or lower it to normal levels.*

Spinal cord *Bundles of nerve fibres run through the centre of the spine carrying impulses between the brain and the body.*

Map of the brain

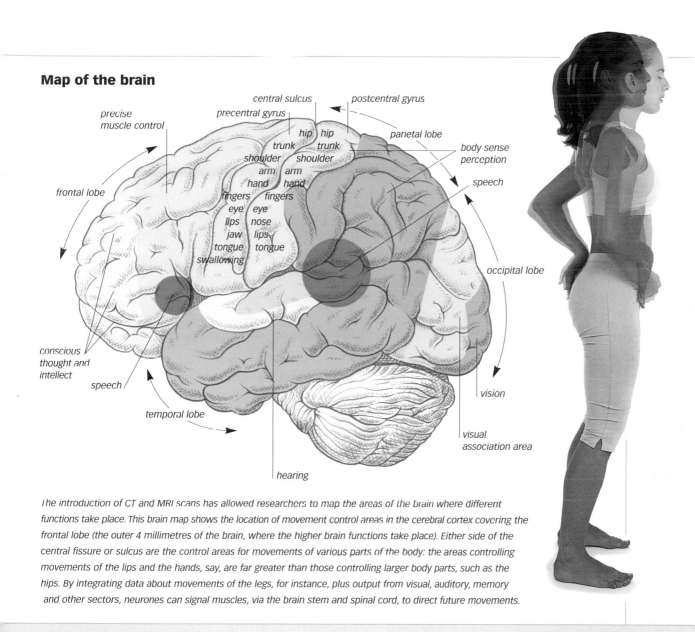

precise muscle control

precentral gyrus

central sulcus

postcentral gyrus

parietal lobe

frontal lobe

hip hip
trunk trunk
shoulder shoulder
arm arm
hand hand
fingers fingers
eye eye
lips nose
jaw lips
tongue tongue
swallowing

body sense perception

speech

occipital lobe

conscious thought and intellect

speech

temporal lobe

hearing

vision

visual association area

The introduction of CT and MRI scans has allowed researchers to map the areas of the brain where different functions take place. This brain map shows the location of movement control areas in the cerebral cortex covering the frontal lobe (the outer 4 millimetres of the brain, where the higher brain functions take place). Either side of the central fissure or sulcus are the control areas for movements of various parts of the body: the areas controlling movements of the lips and the hands, say, are far greater than those controlling larger body parts, such as the hips. By integrating data about movements of the legs, for instance, plus output from visual, auditory, memory and other sectors, neurones can signal muscles, via the brain stem and spinal cord, to direct future movements.

The higher brain centres

The brain consists of grey or white nerve tissue fed by blood and lymph vessels. These supply oxygen, potassium, magnesium and other nutrients the neurones need to operate. Making movements at will involves decision- making in the areas, where conscious thought occurs:

Cerebrum Largest brain area, consists mainly of white matter (bundles of nerve fibres or axons), which provides pathways for nerve impulses travelling to and from the lower brain and the cerebral cortex, which covers the cerebrum.

Cerebral cortex A 4-millimetre-thick layer of grey matter (neurones), seat of the senses, bodily

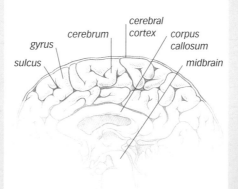

gyrus

sulcus

cerebrum

cerebral cortex

corpus callosum

midbrain

sensation and voluntary movement. Here, the thought-processing centres receive and analyze data from the lower brain centres, from the senses, and from each other, to initiate movements and actions.

Corpus callosum A bridge of white matter connecting the left and right sides of the brain. It provides the largest of the many pathways along which nerve impulses are transmitted from left to right side and back.

Basal ganglia Four islands of grey matter (nuclei and cell bodies of neurones) in the white matter deep in the centre of the cerebrum. They regulate automatic movements, receiving impulses from the brain stem, and communicate via the cerebellum with the postural muscles to fine tune their actions and produce smooth coordination.

37

Understanding reflexes

Touch the palm of a new baby, and the baby grasps the finger tightly. This primitive reflex may have endured from times when infants needed to cling to their mothers for safety. It is one of several reflexes babies develop in the womb for their survival at birth. Another is the suck reflex: touch a baby's cheek and it turns its head in the direction of the touch, making sucking movements. A reflex is an automatic response to stimulation of the body. The knee jerk is a reflex reaction of receptors in the joint to stretching caused when a hammer hits the knee.

Primitive reflexes are only needed for a few months after birth. In the first year, they are normally inhibited by the higher brain centres and replaced by postural reflexes that enable the child to move freely. For example, during its first six months a baby's neck muscles strengthen and it holds up its head. This stimulates organs of orientation in the inner ear, integrating the sense of balance with the sight, sound, and touch. The baby gains a new perception of its position in space relative to objects and people.

Explaining postural problems

Peter Blythe and Sally Goddard at the Institute for Neuro-Physiological Psychology in England discovered that in some children, these primitive reflexes persist after infancy into childhood, and sometimes beyond. We can learn movements only as our brain and nerve network reach their crucial stages of development, but equally, mastering new movements enables brain development to progress. In early life, anything that interferes with normal development will therefore inhibit movement. Starving a fetus of oxygen by smoking during pregnancy, for instance, or as a result of fetal distress during birth, may well inhibit the normal development of movement.

In her book, *A Teacher's Window into the Child's Mind,* Sally Goddard describes how failing to make the transition from primitive to postural reflexes may result in problems such as poor balance and coordination, uneven walking, stooping and clumsiness. The Institute's remedial programmes use a range of techniques, including exercise, to encourage the brain to reinterpret information that initiates the primitive reflex, and so enable individuals to move on to the postural reflex stage.

Achieving structural integration

Generally, exercise can benefit people with balance and coordination problems. It helps them develop new ways of moving and integrates these into the body so they feel and become natural. For instance, stretching and bending while lying on the floor, as in the corkscrew on page 194–95, rolling the hips, as on pages 150–51, and rotations like the Spinal spiral on page 101, all help correct movement and posture imbalances that may relate to the effects of undeveloped reflex responses.

Attaining structural fitness therefore involves regular practice to restore flexibility to a body that has stiffened through disuse, and relearning basic movements. If this sounds like hard work, be reassured that even bouncing on a mini-trampoline is a good way to revise incompletely developed movement patterns – and it is fun. Our lengthening lifespan makes it increasingly necessary to take personal responsibility for maintaining body structure. The body is a machine with a limited timespan, but by caring for its moving parts, we can maintain its performance at optimum levels through its natural life. You are never to old to begin structural fitness.

Babies swim along the birth canal, turning their arms and shoulders. These birthing movements may be essential first stages in a learning pattern for movement. Sitting follows, then crawling, standing and walking. An infant must perfect each step before progressing to the next. Failure to do so may impede development of the brain's motor (movement) centres.

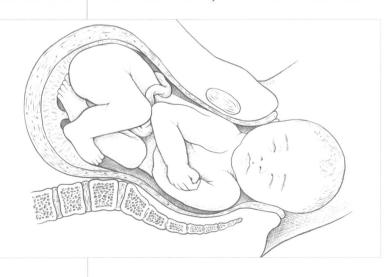

Left brain-right brain

A long fold called the longitudinal fissure divides the brain into left and right hemispheres. The motor nerves leave the left hemisphere, and at the point where they reach the medulla in the brain stem, they cross over those leaving the right hemisphere. The result is that the left side of the brain controls the right side of the body, and the left side of the body is controlled by the right side of the brain.

The two hemispheres are thought to mirror each other at birth, but during early childhood, one hemisphere usually takes over some of the higher functions. In most people, the left hemisphere governs many functions related to language and is said to be dominant, but in others, the right hemisphere governs language abilities. A number of people develop no dominant hemisphere, and this is thought to be related to difficulties with reading, writing and drawing, and poor spatial judgment and orientation. However, people vary enormously in the degree to which one hemisphere is dominant.

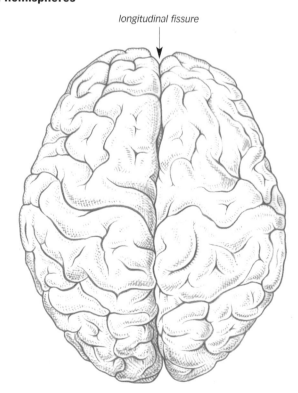

Simply repeating an exercise on one side of the body and then on the other helps you improve on your left-right coordination and balance.

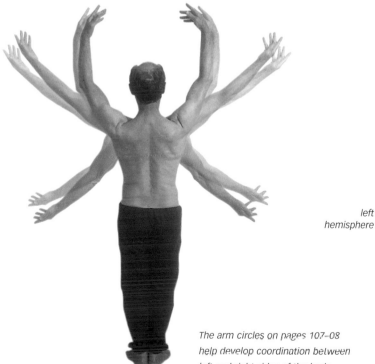

The arm circles on pages 107–08 help develop coordination between left and right sides of the body.

The brain hemispheres

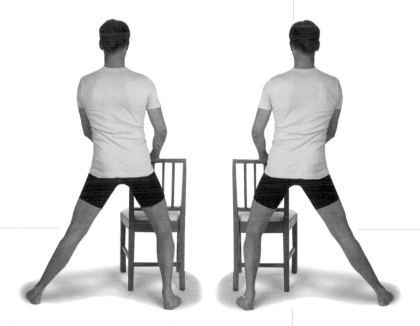

longitudinal fissure

left hemisphere

right hemisphere

part 3
key muscles

There is a pattern in the body, visible in its contours.
We must learn to see it, to know with surety that
a particular contour speaks of underlying elements
fitting together in a certain way.

IDA P. ROLF

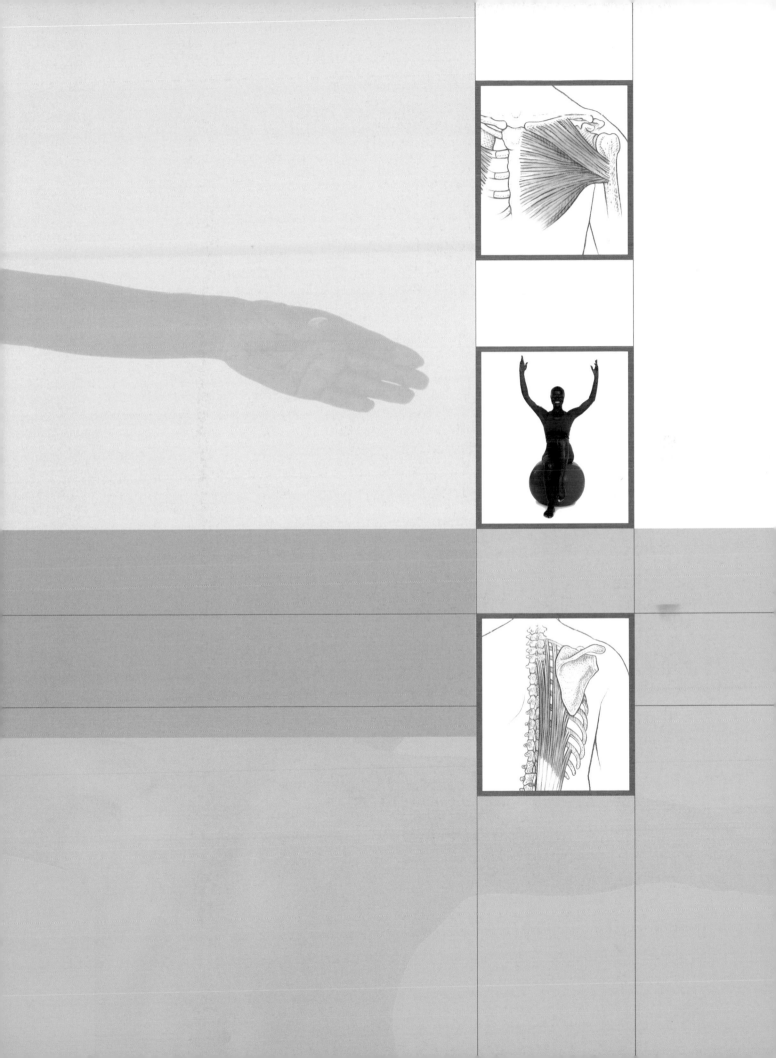

Muscles and movement

Every physical action, from eye-blink to heartbeat, out-breath to high jump, is powered by the contractions of the muscles. Movement is evidence of the efficiency and balance of the muscles as they animate the bones, because muscles and their actions are weakened by inactivity and they can be transformed by exercise and training. To every body builder, sumo wrestler, dancer, gymnast and athlete who has won applause, muscles have meant power. This chapter identifies some of the key muscles whose power give the human body its extraordinary vocabulary of movement.

Anatomists have named some 300 muscles in the body, but many muscles have more than one function. For example, each deltoid muscle turns the arm outwards, but the fibres at the front of the shoulder can act alone to move the arm forwards, and the fibres at the back can act independently to extend it outwards.

The muscles we use to move the bones and other body parts, down to the eyelids, at will, are called skeletal muscles. They are formed from fibres that contract and relax, when stimulated nerve impulses, to pull in and push out, lift and lower. Most skeletal muscles are attached by strong, cordlike tendons to two bones, connected by a joint. Bones, joints and muscles form a system of counterbalancing pulleys and levers, with the joints acting as a fulcrum. This system moves the body parts by pulling and releasing, producing an extraordinary range of movement.

Making muscles move

Some muscles work together, and others in opposition, to bend and extend. As we contract or shorten the quadriceps muscles in the thigh to straighten the leg, the hamstrings at the back of the thigh relax or lengthen. To bend the leg, the opposite happens: the hamstrings shorten and the quadriceps lengthen. These contractions and relaxations occur when the muscle is stimulated by an impulse from the nerve that supplies it.

Most skeletal muscles can move in many directions, and the independent actions of many muscles coordinate to turn, bend, stretch and rotate the neck, trunk and limbs in all directions. Many muscles can wrap obliquely from their point of attachment to a bone, past the joint they move. This enables the limbs and other parts of the body to rotate left and right, allowing very small adjustments in the direction in which, for example, a ball is kicked, a dart is thrown, or a golf swing is followed through.

It is a marvel how the actions of all the muscles involved in complex activities are integrated in a lively way. As we walk, the arms swing in opposition to the legs. The body adjusts its shifting balance against the changing ground, while we look and listen, stop, perhaps, to speak to another person, alter direction to avoid bumping into someone, and suddenly dash across a street.

The aim of exercise is to enable the body to maintain that flexibility and so sustain its full vocabulary of movement as you age. Starting with the neck and finishing at the feet, the following pages explain the actions of the muscles you will be stretching and exercising in Part 5, and explore their actions.

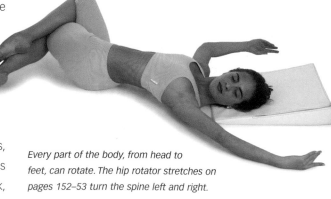

Every part of the body, from head to feet, can rotate. The hip rotator stretches on pages 152–53 turn the spine left and right.

Describing movements

Each part of the body has a different range of movement, and every movement has a name. Here, the models demonstrate some of the body's movement potential.

Extension

These two demonstrators are s-t-r-e-t-c-h-i-n-g out or extending their legs, arms, abdomen, chest and neck. To extend is to move the bones on either side of a joint apart.

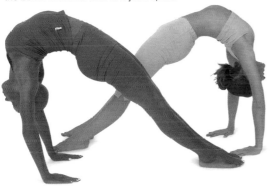

Flexion

To flex part of the body is to bend it, bringing the bones on either side of a joint closer together. This demonstrator is flexing her spine and elbow joints.

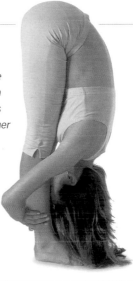

Abduction

This demonstrator is abducting her thigh – or moving it outwards, away from the midline. You can also abduct your arms and shoulders.

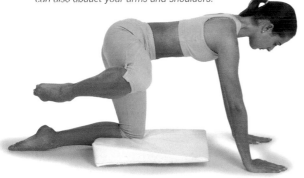

Adduction

The right leg is being adducted here – moving inwards, towards the midline. You can also adduct your arms and shoulders.

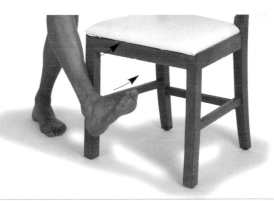

Dorsiflexion

You dorsiflex your hand or foot by pulling it upwards. Dorsiflexion is bending backwards – for the foot it is the opposite of pointing.

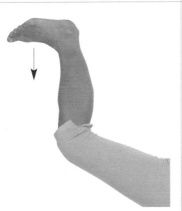

Plantar flexion

Plantar flexion is something your feet do: you extend your ankle joint and raise your heel, standing on tiptoe.

Muscles and exercise

The muscles we use for exercise range from the delicate muscles that control the toes to the large muscles of the back, and their fibres are very different shapes, depending on the amount of force they generate. The strongest muscles are spindle-shaped and have fibres arranged longitudinally; and some, like the biceps, the triceps and the quadriceps in the thigh, divide into two, three or four separately working sets of fibres. Certain types of muscle fibre respond rapidly to stimulation from the nerves that supply them, and others more slowly; while some use the energy more quickly than others and soon tire.

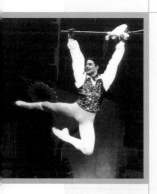

Dancers need to be able to generate short bursts of concentrated energy in order to execute high leaps, yet they also need stamina and endurance. They train every muscle to achieve its full range of movement.

Exercise uses energy, but muscle movements are not powered by heat. Instead, they use chemical energy from glucose, a simple sugar. When food breaks down during digestion, molecules of glucose pass from the stomach into the bloodstream and are carried to every cell in the body. When stimulated by the nerves to provide energy for exercise, however, the muscle cells cannot release energy from the glucose directly. Instead, they couple glucose molecules with molecules of another compound called ATP (adenosine triphosphate). ATP can release energy from glucose molecules in an explosive burst, and the muscle cells can use it to generate movement. Sports scientists call ATP the 'energy currency' of the muscles.

Releasing energy causes ATP to break down into another compound, ADP (adenosine diphosphate). But when the muscle cells use more glucose, the ADP can recombine with its by-products into energy-generating ATP. As scientists unravelled the role of ATP in energy release during the 1960s, the value of a high-carbohydrate diet for sports training became clear, especially for activities such as basketball, which needs short, powerful bursts of energy.

Stamina vs. concentrated energy

Publicity about these discoveries and others, such as the involvement of slow-twitch and fast-twitch muscle fibres in different kinds of exercise, led to the 1980s craze for aerobics – continuous exercise involving sustained high oxygen consumption. Sports scientists found that muscle fibres with a red pigment are suited to aerobic exercise.

They are called slow-twitch fibres because they respond relatively slowly to electrochemical stimulation; but they can resynthesize ATP from ADP, and so tire less easily than fast-twitch fibres. They can sustain long periods of aerobic exercise such as dancing or bouncing on a trampoline.

White muscle fibres are called fast-twitch fibres because they contract quickly when stimulated by nerves. They generate energy rapidly for fast, powerful activities, such as the final sprint in a race, or a goal strike in a football match, but tire quickly. One type of fast-twitch fibre can withstand longer periods of aerobic activity, and another responds faster to anaerobic demands.

People generally have around 50% slow-twitch and 50% fast-twitch fibres in the muscles of their legs and arms. However, long-distance runners, cross-country skiers, canoeists, distance swimmers, and other endurance athletes may have as much as 90% of slow-twitch fibres in their key muscles, while sprinters and team sport players have a higher proportion of fast-twitch fibres. Javelin and discus throwers, long and high jumpers, and martial artists have a more equal distribution.

In time, exercise training seems to alter the relative proportions of fast- and slow-twitch fibres in the muscles. Future research may show that this is the end effect of structural fitness exercises, which seek to ensure that all muscles achieve their full range of movement. All sports are one-sided, over-exercising certain muscles, and in specific directions only, and structural fitness exercises aim to restore balance. They increase blood and oxygen flow to all muscles, maximizing their range of movement.

The anatomy of a muscle

The muscles you can move at will are the skeletal muscles, so called because they are attached to two or more bones, which they move. A muscle has a belly of long fibres wrapped in a sheath of connective tissue. A nerve stimulus causes a chemical change in the muscle, which makes its fibres relax or lengthen, as illustrated on the right, or contract or shorten, as shown far right.

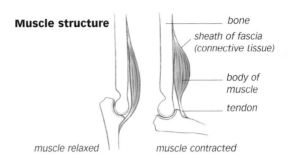

Muscle structure

- bone
- sheath of fascia (connective tissue)
- body of muscle
- tendon

muscle relaxed　　　*muscle contracted*

Origin and insertion points

Skeletal muscles are wrapped in connective tissue, and this forms a strong, elastic tendon at either end. Each tendon is normally attached to a different bone, one of which remains almost stationary and the other is moved when the muscle contracts or shortens. By tradition, the point at which the tendon attaches to the stationary bone is called the 'origin' and the attachment to the bone that moves is called the 'insertion'. The humerus in the shoulder is the origin of the biceps muscle in the upper arm, and its insertion point is the radius in the forearm, just below the elbow joint.

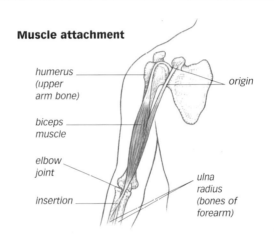

Muscle attachment

- humerus (upper arm bone)
- origin
- biceps muscle
- elbow joint
- insertion
- ulna radius (bones of forearm)

Agonists and antagonists

Pairs and groups of skeletal muscles work together to produce smoothly coordinated movement. When a pair of muscles works together, the muscle that initiates the movement is called the 'agonist', and the muscle that opposes it, the 'antagonist'. When you raise your forearm, the agonist is the biceps muscle, which contracts to pull the forearm upward. The antagonist is the triceps muscle, which relaxes. To lower the forearm, the triceps becomes the agonist and contracts, while the biceps acts as the antagonist by relaxing. When a group of muscles acts in unison, the one that initiates the action is called the 'prime mover' and the other muscles that contribute to the action are called 'synergists'.

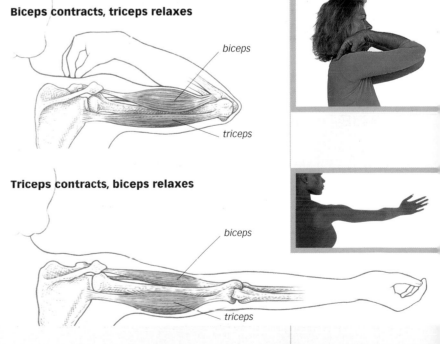

Biceps contracts, triceps relaxes

- biceps
- triceps

Triceps contracts, biceps relaxes

- biceps
- triceps

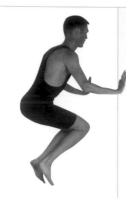

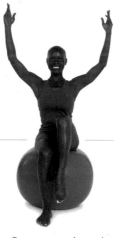

Muscle structure

The fibres of skeletal muscles look like long strands bundled together.

The strands range in length from less than 2 millimetres ($^1/_{10}$th of an inch) in the smallest muscles, such as those that execute the fine movements of the fingers, to 30 centimetres (12 inches) in the longest, such as the sartorius in the leg.

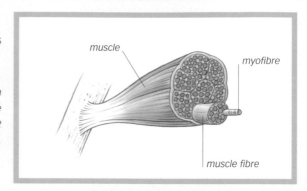

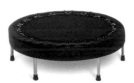
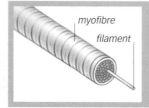
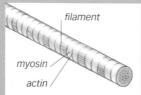
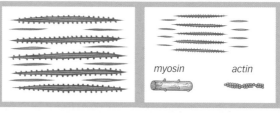

The bundles consist of cylinder-shaped cells called myofibres.

The myofibres consist of two types of fine filament, which overlap. The thicker filaments are called 'myosin' and the thinner 'actin'.

Seen through a microscope, muscle tissue is striped. The light bands are actin filaments and the dark bands are where actin and myosin filaments overlap slightly.

When a nerve stimulates a muscle fibre, the actin and myosin filaments slide right over each other. This shortens each myofibre, reducing the lengths of the muscle fibre bundles, and so shortening the muscle.

Everyone needs regular aerobic exercise to strengthen the heart and lungs and increase the oxygen content of the blood. Low-impact aerobic exercises on a bouncer (top) or an exercise ball (above) make an ideal partnership with pilates.

Muscle fatigue

Muscles tire if used repeatedly without adequate rest. During anaerobic exercise, the cells' reserves of ATP quickly become depleted. In aerobic exercise a point is reached when the blood cannot supply nutrients such as oxygen as fast as they are being used, and the cells have to generate energy without using oxygen. This produces lactic acid. This chemical cannot be removed as quickly as it is produced, so it accumulates in the cells, causing loss of muscle tension.

Aerobic exercise depletes the body's reserves of glucose so that the muscles eventually become fatigued.

The body could mobilize stores of lipids or fats in the liver and tissues to supply energy, but when the muscles' glucose reserves are lowered, the muscle cells tire despite having plenty of oxygen, and they are unable to mobilize energy reserves in the liver and fat tissues.

Regular training improves the endurance of muscles by increasing the number of blood vessels, enabling

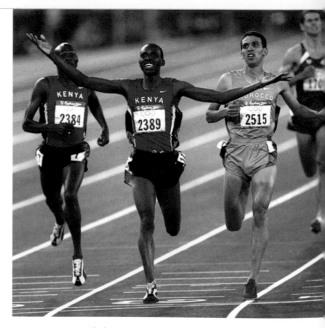

more oxygen and glucose to reach the muscle cells more rapidly, speeding and prolonging the production of ATP so that it becomes possible to exercise vigorously for longer without tiring.

Muscle action

The main purpose of the pilates system is to maintain the natural functioning of the body's systems, and its aim in exercising the muscles is to restore their efficiency and maintain their full range of movement. This has a bonus in improving appearance, for the shape of the body is largely determined by its muscle structure. When the muscles are fully developed, working correctly, and in balance, the proportions of the whole body look right. The following pages locate and identify the body's key muscles and illustrate their range of actions.

The upper body

The collar-bones at the front and the shoulder blades at the back are the struts on which the movements of head, neck, and shoulders depend. They provide the main anchor points for the major muscles that move the skull, the uppermost vertebrae of the spine, the shoulders, and the arms. They are extremely mobile – the shoulder blades move smoothly up and down, left and right – giving head, neck, and shoulders great freedom of movement. Eight muscles of the shoulder girdle are attached both to the shoulder blades and to the humerus, the bone of the upper arm. They include the great muscles of the chest and back, pectoralis

major and latissimus dorsi, the deltoid and supraspinatus, and a group of smaller muscles whose job is to rotate the upper arm. These muscles need to be relaxed, but strong enough to move the arms, and stable but mobile so they work together in balance. The trapezius, the rhomboids, the levator scapulae, the serratus anterior, and the pectoralis minor, illustrated on the following pages, stabilize the shoulder blades or scapulae, holding them in place against the thorax. They have a key role in maintaining the correct posture of the head, upper body and cervical spine, and the alignment of the whole body takes its cue from them.

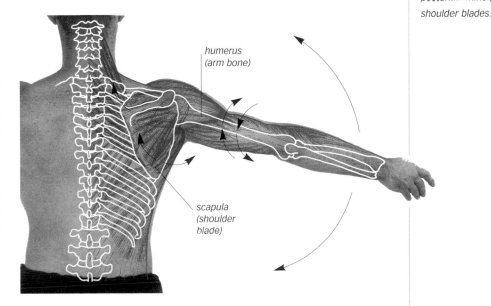

Massage and exercise help straighten rounded shoulders. If you tend to hunch them, your shoulder blades become rigid. The back of your head tilts back and your chin rises, blocking the movements of the atlas and axis and so restricting head movements. The upper spine curves. Massage releases tension in the trapezius, the rhomboids, the serratus anterior, and the pectoralis minor, freeing the shoulder blades.

The muscles that move the arm and shoulder are attached to the borders and spine of the scapulae or shoulder blades, positioning them against the ribs. The scapulae are very mobile, gliding over the ribs when the arms are flexed and extended. The shoulder blades and humerus (upper arm bone) move together in a 'scapulohumeral rhythm': the humerus describes a large arc at the shoulder joint, while the shoulder blade describes a small arc as it rotates over the ribs. To raise your arms above your head while keeping your shoulders down, you must rotate your arm in its socket. If the joint is inflamed, as in frozen shoulder, or the muscles stiff, you cannot lift your arms without raising your shoulders.

humerus
(arm bone)

scapula
(shoulder
blade)

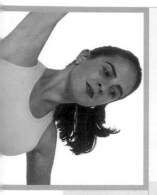

Postural muscles of the neck

These muscles raise, lower and rotate the head and neck. They consist of deep muscles, attached to the upper cervical vertebrae, that work with more superficial muscles such as the trapezius, the sternomastoid and the prevertebral muscles (see below) to control the position of the head as it lifts from a prone position and to keep it level when moving. The proprioceptors or sensors in these muscles signal the position of the head to the brain. The scalenus medius also assists in breathing by lifting the upper ribs.

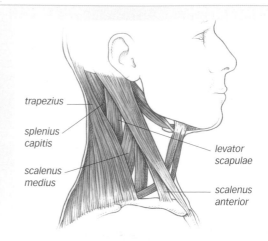

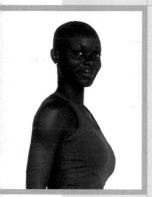

Sternocleidomastoid

Turn your head and neck to one side and the sternocleidomastoid becomes visible, forming a ridge down the opposite side of the neck between the sternum (breastbone) and the clavicle (collar-bone) to the mastoid process behind the ear. Its origin and insertion points give this muscle its name, which is usually shortened to 'sternomastoid'. The left sternomastoid tilts the head left and turns the face to the right, and its partner on the right tilts the head to the right and turns the face to the left. Together they flex the neck forward, help to lift the head from a prone position, and to rotate it, and help elevate the upper ribs during breathing.

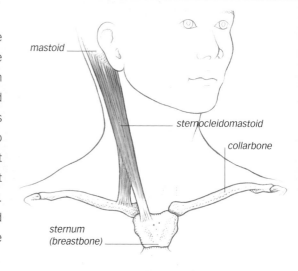

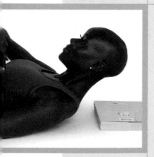

Prevertebral muscles

These muscles work with the postural muscles and the sternomastoid (above) to flex or bend the head on the neck, and to flex the neck forward and lift it. If they are weak you have no control over the orientation and placing of your head if you try to lift it when lying down. The head and neck exercises in Level 1 work these muscles against gravity while you are standing, and the Level 3 exercises strengthen them by making you coordinate the movements of your head and body while working on the mat.

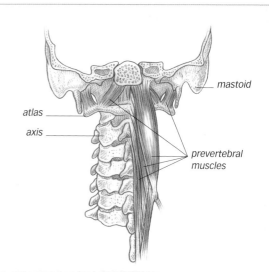

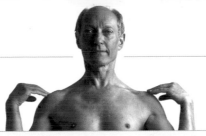

Trapezius

This trapezium-shaped outer muscle of the shoulder girdle has two sections. The upper fibres originate in the skull and insert into the collar-bone and the shoulder blade; they pull both up and rotate the shoulder blade outward. The lower fibres originate in the spine and insert into the spine of the shoulder blade to pull it down. They work together with the rhomboids (below) to pull the shoulder blades to the spine when standing to attention, to raise the arms above the head, and to rotate them back and forwards as in rowing. They also help the sternomastoid turn the head.

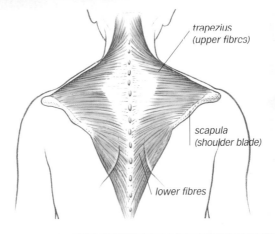

trapezius (upper fibres)

scapula (shoulder blade)

lower fibres

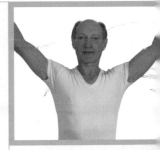

The rhomboids and levator scapulae

The rhomboids major and minor and the levator scapulae are the principal muscles responsible for pulling the shoulder blades back towards the spine, and rotating them outwards. They are deep muscles, originating in the lower cervical and the thoracic vertebrae, and inserting into the borders of the shoulder blades. The rhomboids work with the trapezius to pull the shoulder blades back towards the spine in the military stance. They act in opposition to the serratus anterior (see below), the muscle that lies directly over them. The levator scapulae pull the shoulder blades upwards, so they assist the movements of the arms.

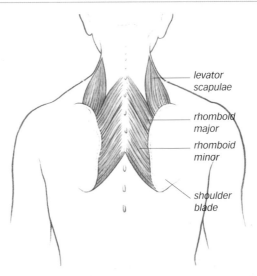

levator scapulae

rhomboid major

rhomboid minor

shoulder blade

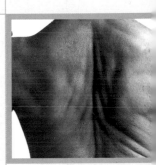

Serratus anterior

This is the muscle you use when you brush your hair, and it keeps the shoulder blades in place when you carry a heavy suitcase. It consists of a thin sheet of muscle, extending from its origin at the side of the chest in the first eight ribs, to its insertion in the shoulder blades at the back (shown in the illustration). The serratus anterior is sometimes called the fencer's muscle because its principal function is to pull the shoulder blades round the chest from the back to the front when stretching and reaching. If the two serratus anterior muscles become stiff and immobile, they fail to keep the shoulder blades in place against the ribs, which then stand out like wings, especially when the arms are raised. They work with the trapezius to rotate the shoulder blades outwards.

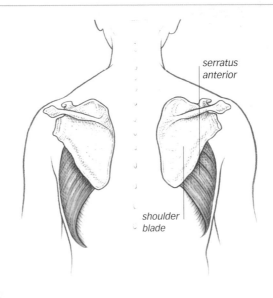

serratus anterior

shoulder blade

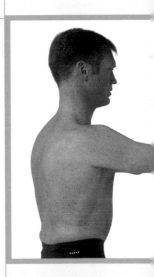

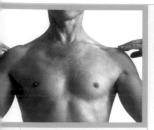

The pectorals

These hardworking muscles (often called 'the pecs) adduct and flex the arm and rotate it towards the centre of the body. Body builders pump iron to make the pectoralis major bulge impressively. This 'great chest muscle' adducts the arms, but the upper fibres, originating on the collar-bone and attached to the upper humerus, can act separately to pull the arm up; and the lower fibres, attached to the breastbone and upper ribs, push it out. Pectoralis minor is one of the stabilizers of the shoulder blades. It originates on the third, fourth, and fifth ribs and inserts into the shoulder blade to draw it forward and down. These muscles can also lift and lower the ribs to aid breathing.

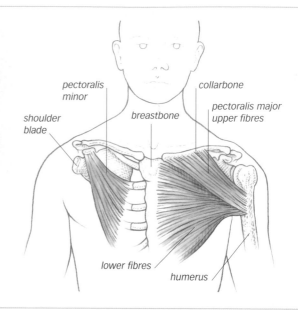

Deltoid and supraspinatus

The deltoid and supraspinatus work together to abduct the shoulder – move it out and back. The supraspinatus is a small muscle, originating at the top of the shoulder blade, with its tendon inserted into the shoulder joint. It works against gravity to start the abduction movement, for the deltoid to take over. The deltoid looks like a shoulder pad and shapes the shoulder. The front fibres originate in the collar-bone and insert into the humerus, and act alone to flex the arm forwards. At the back, the posterior fibres, shown in the illustration, which originate in the spine of the shoulder blade and insert into the humerus, extend the arm out to the side.

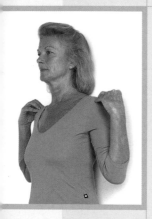

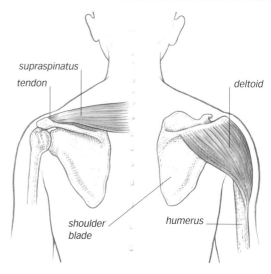

Biceps brachii and the triceps

The biceps stretches from its origin in the shoulder blade to its insertion in the radius, the large bone of the forearm. This is the strong muscle that bends the elbow, and it also rotates the forearm into the palms-up position. It works in opposition to the triceps, the muscle that does all the work when you want to extend the elbow joint to straighten your arm. The triceps also originates in the shoulder blade, but it inserts in the ulna, the smaller of the two bones of the forearm. These are complex muscles, as their names imply: the biceps divides into two heads, each with a separate origin; and the triceps divides into three heads with separate origin points.

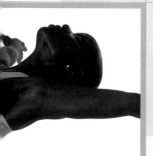

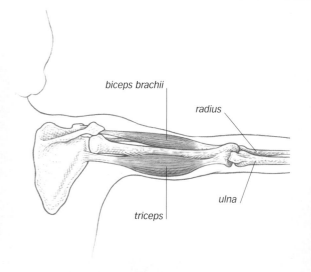

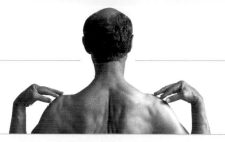

The spine and back

Well over 100 pairs of muscles support the spine, and flex, extend, and rotate it in all directions. Shown below are the erector spinae, which support the vertebrae, keeping them in position. The scalenus, intertransversarii, and rotatores muscle groups, deeply located on the bony projections of the vertebrae, are composed of small muscles, each one connecting a few vertebrae. Together they lift the trunk and flex and rotate the

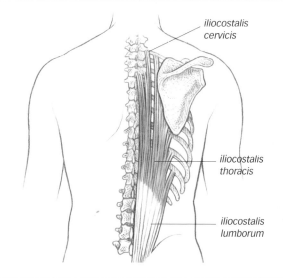

spine. Their concerted movements contribute to the stronger actions of the larger deep muscles of the lower back. These postural muscles ceaselessly adjust the body to counter gravity. If they are allowed to weaken, the posture and alignment of upper and lower body suffer.

Each one of the muscles that move the spine has a very limited range of motion, but all work together to give the back its remarkable flexibility.

Erector spinae

These muscles keep the spine upright and stretch it up. 'Erector spinae' is a collective name for several muscle groups. For example, at the base of the spine is the iliocostalis lumborum group, which inserts into the sacrum and extends, abducts and rotates the lumbar spine. The iliocostalis thoracis group in the middle and the iliocostalis cervicis, which originates in the first six ribs and inserts into the vertebrae of the upper back and neck, stretch the spine up. The multifidus group (see page 155) are also erector spinae. They are deep muscles that rotate, stretch and flex the lower back. Semispinalis capitis is a deep neck muscle that bends the head to one side.

iliocostalis
cervicis

iliocostalis
thoracis

iliocostalis
lumborum

The rotator muscles

The rotatores are a group of small muscles, each located on one of the bony side projections, called transverse processes, of a vertebra, and connected to the vertebra above it. Their concerted action rotates the body to the opposite side. They work in tandem with the multifidus (see page 155), a group of larger muscles, each spanning two to four vertebrae from their origin in the sacrum to the thoracic vertebrae of the upper back. Both sets of rotatores and multifidus muscles on either side of the spine work together to stretch the whole trunk; while those on the left work together to rotate the trunk to the right, and vice versa.

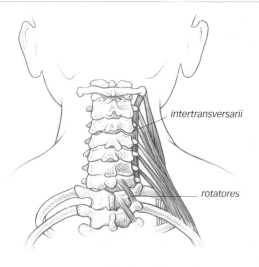

intertransversarii

rotatores

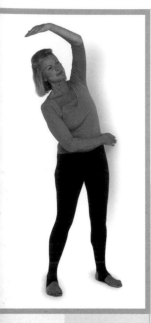

Quadratus lumborum

This is sometimes called the 'lower back muscle' because it bends the lumbar spine. It is a deep muscle, originating at the top of the pelvic bone and inserting into the 12th (floating) rib, which it fixes in position. It is involved in breathing, since it pulls the 12th rib downwards, enabling the diaphragm to lower, drawing air into the lungs. The action of each muscle in the pair can be reversed voluntarily to lift each hip independently.

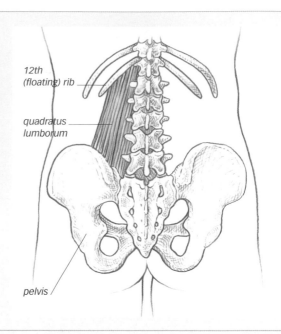

12th (floating) rib

quadratus lumborum

pelvis

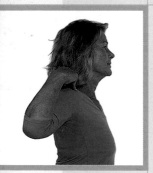

Latissimus dorsi

These large muscles cover most of the back. They originate at the spine, on ribs 9 to 12, the shoulder blade, and the pelvis, and their insertion points are in the humerus. If the arms are anchored they pull the whole body up to the arms – so these are the muscles you use to do pull-ups. They also help pull back the arm for archery, and archery will develop these muscles. The latissimus dorsi assist in breathing by squeezing the rib cage when you breathe out.

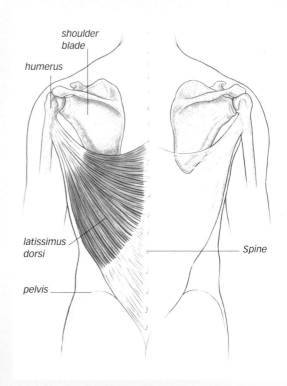

shoulder blade

humerus

latissimus dorsi

pelvis

Spine

The abdomen

Four large muscles wrap around the abdomen like a corset, supporting and cushioning the internal organs, holding them in place. They help bend the trunk forwards and sideways, rotate it, and tilt the pelvis. Tightening them creates pressure in the abdomen. It is needed for coughing, defecating, and childbirth, but prolonged, habitual tightening can deepen the low back curve. When strong and elastic, these muscles maintain good posture by keeping this curve shallow and the pelvis correctly aligned.

Rectus abdominis

This muscle shows up as the 'six pack' in men when it is developed. In fact, it is two long muscles, their fibres running side by side up the abdomen from their origin in the pubic bone to their insertion in the xiphoid process of the breastbone (see page 96) and ribs 5, 6 and 7. Bands of tough connective tissue divide each muscle into three segments, forming the 'six pack', and connective tissue called the rectus sheath covers them. This muscle flexes the trunk, pulling the lower body toward the rib cage. You use it when, lying prone, you lift your shoulders or legs.

External and internal obliques

The external obliques descend from the ribs to the pubic bone and wrap around the sides of the abdomen. They work with the smaller internal obliques beneath them, and with the rectus abdominis, to flex or bend the trunk. Their fibres angle downwards, so the obliques on the left bend and rotate the trunk to the left, and the right obliques bend and rotate it to the right. Touch your left foot with your right hand, and you use the right external oblique and the left internal oblique to flex and twist the trunk.

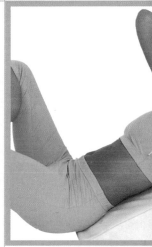

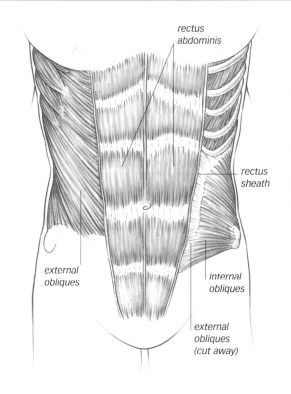

rectus abdominis

rectus sheath

external obliques

internal obliques

external obliques (cut away)

Transversus abdominis

These two muscles lie in the abdomen's muscular wall, beneath the rectus abdominis and the internal obliques. Their fibres cross the abdomen. They originate in the lower six ribs and the top of the hip bone and insert into the linea alba, the strip of connective tissue along the midline of the abdomen. They hold the internal organs in place and, by balancing the action of the muscles of the pelvic floor (see pages 129–34), prevent them from sagging. Structural fitness depends on maintaining good elasticity and tone in these important muscles.

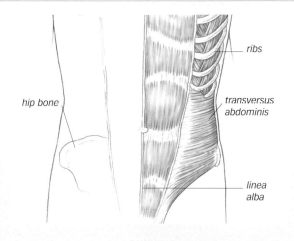

ribs

hip bone

transversus abdominis

linea alba

The lower body

The internal and external muscles of the abdomen, hips and thighs work together, agonists and antagonists imposing equal resistance to keep the upper and lower body in alignment. What is often forgotten is that to keep structurally fit, these muscles must be stretched as well as contracted.

A weak or undeveloped muscle in the group causes the rectus abdominis to pull the balance of the body forwards. If key muscles of the hips and thighs, such as the iliopsoas and the hamstrings, are regularly stretched, they can counter this tendency by pulling the pelvis upright.

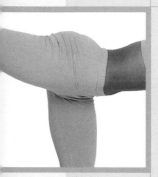

The gluteals

Exercise your gluteal muscles to keep your seat firm and trim. Gluteus maximus, the outer buttock muscle, extends the thigh, contracting to straighten it as when rising from sitting to standing, and relaxes when the body is upright. It also belongs to the muscle group that rotates the thigh laterally. The smaller gluteus medius, and the gluteus minimus, the innermost muscle of the triad (illustrated below right), abduct the thigh. The front fibres of gluteus medius also adduct it, or rotate it toward the midline of the body, while the posterior fibres abduct it, or rotate it outward. During walking, these two muscles act with the tensor fasciae latae (see page 56) to pull the trunk over the moving leg. This positions the body's centre of gravity over the foot hitting the ground, ready for the trailing foot to take another step.

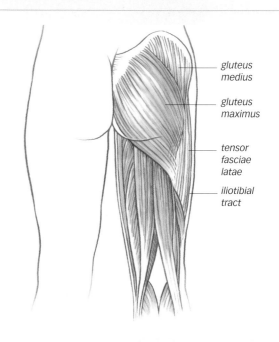

gluteus medius

gluteus maximus

tensor fasciae latae

iliotibial tract

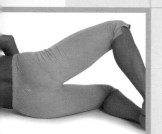

Lateral rotators of the hips

Underneath the buttock muscles a group of six deep muscles links the sacrum, the hip joint, and the head of the thigh bone. With the gluteals they open the hips and rotate the hips and thighs. A lifestyle of sitting, standing and minimal walking tightens the hip rotators, creating an imbalance, particularly of the piriformis. This muscle originates in the sacrum and inserts into the highest point of the femur or thigh bone, and several important nerves pass through it. If tight, it can trap the sciatic nerve. All these muscles need to be stretched to even their balance.

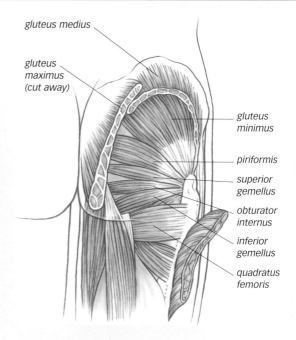

gluteus medius

gluteus maximus (cut away)

gluteus minimus

piriformis

superior gemellus

obturator internus

inferior gemellus

quadratus femoris

The hip flexors

The iliopsoas is the collective name for two muscles: the psoas major and the iliacus, but they are collectively called 'the psoas'. They are the principal hip flexors, essential to the internal stabilizing balance of the lower body. They are deep muscles: psoas major originates on the lumbar vertebrae and iliacus inserts into the femur or thigh bone, so the psoas forms a bridge between trunk and legs. It straightens the thigh and adducts the hip joint – rotating the thigh inward. It connects with the nerves of the lumbar spine, which control the functioning of the viscera, and keeps the pelvis upright and level at the hip joints. To do this effectively it must be strong and flexible, but if it is repeatedly contracted without stretching, it becomes over-taut. This increases the lumbar curve and tilts the pelvis forward, pushing the abdomen outward. The abdominal muscles shorten, pulling down the breastbone and disturbing the carriage of the neck.

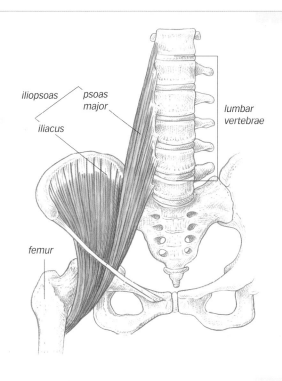

iliopsoas

psoas major

iliacus

lumbar vertebrae

femur

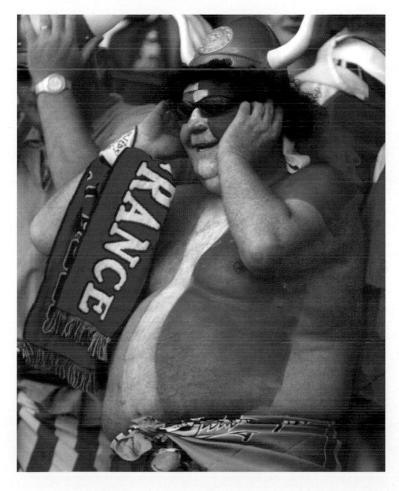

Poor posture and neglecting exercise cause slackening in the tension of the psoas, and this is a major cause of a pot belly. Yet some forms of exercise can have the same effect. Sit-ups carried out with the feet against the floor and the knees bent, tighten and shorten the psoas, making it pull against the lower back and the inside of the thigh bone at the hip. This tilts the stomach forwards, causing it to protrude. One remedy for a pot belly is to stretch the psoas (see page 156).

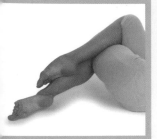

Tensor fasciae latae

This muscle tenses or pulls on the fascia lata (the connective tissue 'stocking' encircling the thigh (see page 31). The tensor fasciae latae originates at the hip and inserts into the iliotibial tract, a thick connective tissue band that runs down the outside of the thigh to the tibia. The gluteus maximus (see page 56) pulls on the iliotibial tract laterally, so when you contract the gluteus maximus and the tensor fasciae latae together, you straighten your knee. The tensor fasciae latae is also one of the muscles that abduct and rotate the hip.

The adductors

The four adductors move the thigh towards the midline of the body. They originate at the pelvis and insert into the thigh bone. Gracilis is an exception. A long, thin muscle, it inserts into the tibia in the leg and helps straighten the knee. These muscles bring the legs side-by-side and cross one thigh over another. Horse riders use them to keep the thighs pressed tightly against the saddle.

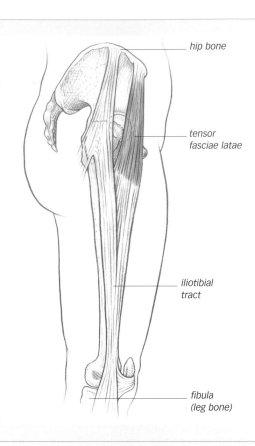

hip bone

tensor fasciae latae

iliotibial tract

fibula (leg bone)

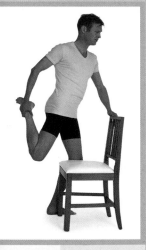

The quadriceps

The quadriceps femoris (called the 'quads') in the thigh is one muscle with four heads. Each has a separate origin – the rectus femoris in the hip and the vastus lateralis, medialis, and intermedius in the femur (thigh bone), so they are treated as four muscles. All insert into the tendon attached to the underside of the kneecap, however. A ligament attaches the kneecap to the tibia, enabling all four muscles to work in unison to extend or straighten the knee. The kneecap slides up, down and sideways over the knee joint when the leg is straightened (see page 123). But when the quads are tightened, the kneecap helps to lock the knee. The rectus femoris also acts on the hip joint to raise the thigh towards the hip.

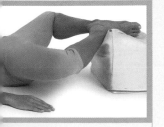

Sartorius

The tailor's muscle, sartorius, stretches diagonally across the front of the thigh from the outside of the pelvis to the inside of the tibia. It flexes the hip and knee joints and rotates the thigh into the crossed-legged position traditionally adopted by tailors.

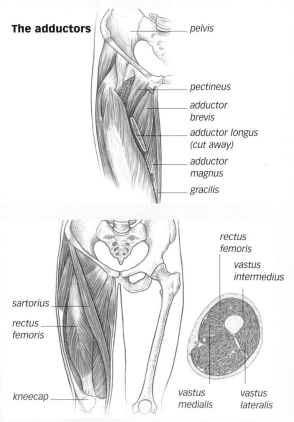

The adductors

pelvis

pectineus

adductor brevis

adductor longus (cut away)

adductor magnus

gracilis

rectus femoris

vastus intermedius

sartorius

rectus femoris

vastus medialis

vastus lateralis

kneecap

The hamstrings

These three muscles have very long tendons and impressive names: the biceps femoris, semitendinosus, and semimembranosus. They stretch from the base of the pelvic girdle, down the thigh, to the tibia and fibula below the knee joint They extend or straighten the hip joint and bend the knee. If their tendons (the 'hamstrings') are not stretched regularly, they shorten and tighten. This is why people who neglect to exercise may find it very painful to bend forwards with the knees straightened, and impossible to touch the toes. Starting a vigorous sport such as football or martial arts without first having stretched and toned the hamstrings makes them vulnerable to damage when kicking.

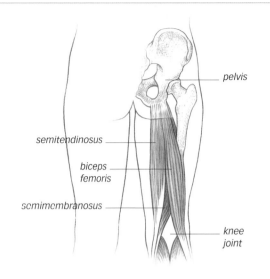

pelvis

semitendinosus

biceps femoris

semimembranosus

knee joint

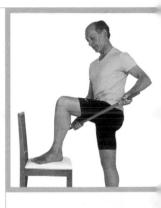

Calf muscles

Stand on tip-toe and gastrocnemius is outlined at the back of the leg, and soleus at the front. These muscles, which shape the lower leg, work as one strong muscle to plantar flex the ankle (see page 43 for plantar flexion). Gastrocnemius originates in the head of the femur at the front of the leg, and soleus in the tibia and fibula – the bones of the leg, but both insert into the Achilles tendon. Gastrocnemius, which moves the knee joint, is more important in running and rapid movement; and soleus stabilizes the ankle joint when standing.

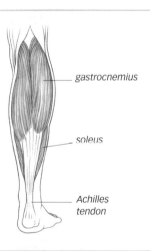

gastrocnemius

soleus

Achilles tendon

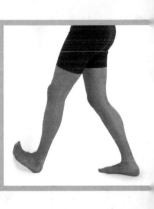

Stirrup muscles

Your feet adjust to uneven surfaces as you walk because the peroneus longus and brevis and the tibialis anterior and posterior work together to invert them (turn them inwards) and evert them (turn them outwards). Osteopaths call these the stirrup muscles because their tendons look like a stirrup beneath each foot, stretching across the middle of the transverse arch.

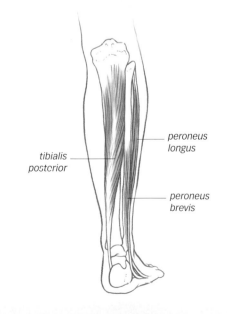

tibialis posterior

peroneus longus

peroneus brevis

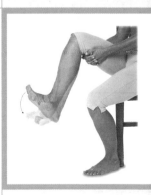

part 4
preparation

Balance reveals the flow of gravitational
energy through the body. Asymmetry
and randomness betray lack of support
by the gravitational field.

IDA P. ROLF

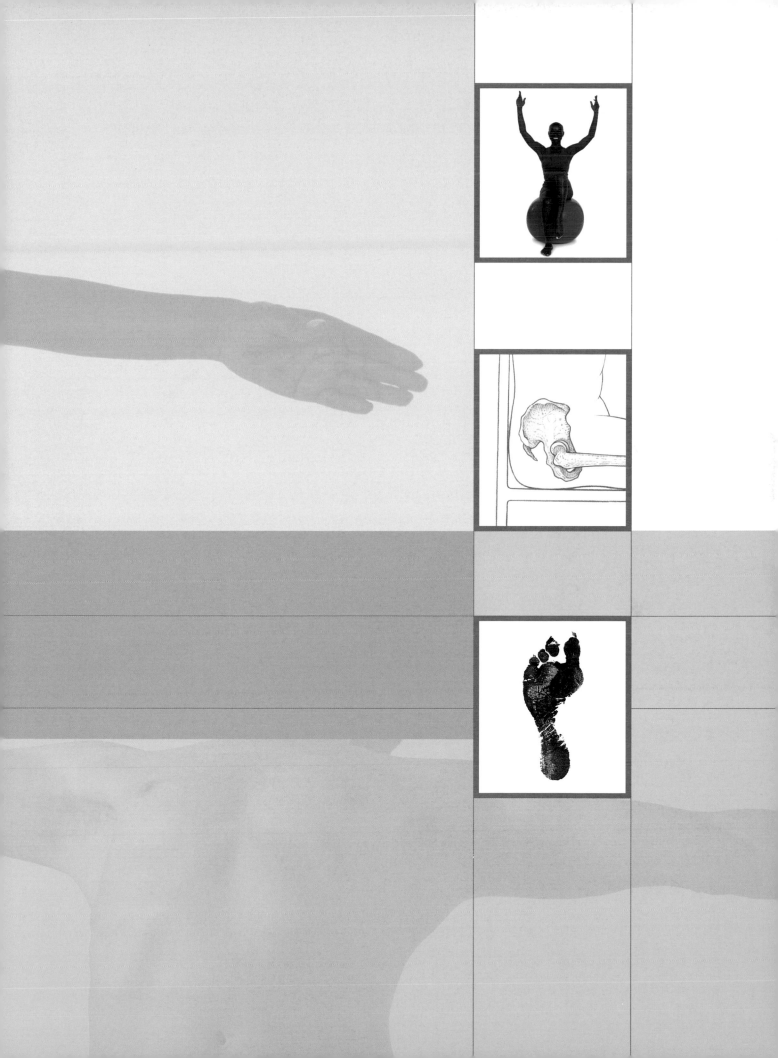

Lifestyle and the body

People give different reasons for wanting to begin pilates exercise. Some have heard it is calming. Others are looking for something they can do alone at home. Many want a less vigorous form of exercise than jogging. These are good reasons for starting, but the best is that the body needs to exercise. Muscles and joints that are not moved and used weaken and deteriorate. Walking for half an hour a day keeps feet, ankles, legs and knees strong, the heart exercised, and the breathing and blood circulation boosted. Exercising for an hour every other day works the whole body, stretching, toning and strengthening every muscle. The bonus is that it leaves you feeling energized.

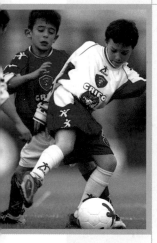

Children and teenagers, whose bodies are still forming and might be damaged by excessive pressure on the joints, may practise pilates but should do so only under expert supervision. Not until the late teens, after the growth spurt of puberty is well advanced, is it wise to practise pilates alone.

Industrialized countries have medical services and an awareness of dietary needs that should have us all brimming with energy. Diseases born of deprivation have been virtually banished. Yet affluence has its health downside: too much comfort and easy transportation seem to discourage people from walking and exercise. Plentiful, varied food leads to overeating and obesity. Overabundant leisure and pleasure seem to result in stress and in futile attempts to counter its effects through smoking, alcoholism, and other recreational drugs.

Medicine and alternative therapies can only alleviate the symptoms of a lifestyle at odds with the body's basic needs, and since the 1970s, educational campaigns by health organizations backed by sports personalities have raised awareness of the dangers of sedentary living. Some people, sensitive to their body's signals, seek to change their sedentary habits and start regular exercise, while signs of impending illness force others to change diet and lifestyle. Health and fitness are now a priority.

Health vs. fitness

Oddly, because the dictionary defines 'fitness' as 'in good health', the two are not synonymous. 'Good health' means 'having no illness'. 'Fitness' has a wider meaning. Professional athletes, dancers, performers and manual workers may work while suffering from sprains, pulled muscles, and fevers – medically, they are ill, yet they are fit enough to carry on their trade. Office workers, by contrast, may rarely be so unfit as to need time off work.

The demands of their jobs rarely cause them physical injury. But are they fit enough to sprint down a road? If they sit at a desk almost all day and they do not exercise regularly, they are not.

Athletics, the marathon, tennis and swimming each works the body in a different way, and each has different fitness requirements. General fitness, to benefit general health, covers levels of cardiovascular endurance, muscle strength and stamina, and flexibility, which are particular to each individual. That most people want to enjoy all-round health and fitness is reflected in the health reasons they give for wanting to start pilates exercises. They want to get rid of recurring back pain, prevent osteoporosis, or reverse the effects that sitting in front of a computer all day is having on their posture.

Making the transition from a no-exercise lifestyle to superfitness level can seem unachievable. Many people try one fitness regime after another, never progressing very far with any, but research shows that keeping up one modest exercise habit, such as going for a moderate daily walk, can transform life expectancy dramatically, no matter what your age or state of health when you begin. For example, people with balance, dizziness or respiratory problems who find it uncomfortable to exercise lying down can practise wall exercises sitting or standing up and improve their balance or lung function. After only ten pilates sessions fairly closely spaced you feel and look better. This chapter explores what pilates involves and what benefits it can bring to mind and body.

QUESTIONNAIRE

Many fitness instructors give new students a questionnaire to complete when they apply to join a pilates studio or class. Here is a self-assessment questionnaire to photocopy and fill in if you are going to work through the exercises in this book alone at home. It will help you decide how best to fit them into your life.

1 Why do I want to learn pilates now?

2 What do I expect to achieve?

3 When am I going to practise?
Note: draw up a schedule of practice times.

4 Where am I going to practise?
Note: turn to pages 14–15 for guidelines.

5 Am I prepared to commit long-term to a discipline that belongs entirely to me and that will fulfil my need to do something entirely for myself?

6 Will this affect my friends/boyfriend or girlfriend/family? In what ways?

Injury and illness

Some people take up exercise hoping it will cure minor aches and pains or help them recover from illness or injury. Pilates exercises can reduce back pain and speed recovery from minor injuries. However, it is sensible to consult a physician and/or a physiotherapist first. If you intend to learn alone, ask a physician to assess your condition. Fill in this questionnaire and take it along to both consultations.

1a Do I have any pain?
Note: how long have I had it? Where? What makes it worse or better? Have I already seen a medical specialist about it?

1b Can I think of any incident or factor – in the past, at work, at home, while driving or cycling or doing any sport or other activity – that might have set off this problem?

2 Have I had any operations? What were they, and when?

3 Have I had any serious falls or other injuries? Any whiplash injury affecting the neck?

4 Do I have any conditions for which I take regular medication?

5 What physical activities have I done in the past for sport and health?

6 What do I do for exercise daily or weekly?

7 Do I have any pain or other symptoms while or after exercising?

8 Have I had a vision test recently?
Note: Uncorrected visual defects may affect the posture of sighted people. Have your eyesight tested and wear glasses or lenses if you need them. Blind and visually impaired people can practise pilates but need to be advised and supervised by a qualified pilates teacher.

Dynamic posture

The first thing a teacher does upon meeting a new client is assess the person's body balance simply by observing posture. Posture is the linchpin of structural balance, so the basic picture of a person's weaknesses, imbalances, and most urgent exercise needs is right there in front of the teacher's eyes before the client's aims, expectations, medical history, aches and pains are detailed. These pages explore body posture and alignment and show how lifestyle and bad posture affect movement and gait, and can, in time, distort the body permanently.

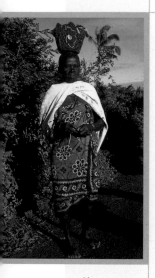

You can carry something heavy on your head if you have good body alignment and posture. Children in African cultures practise from an early age.

Awareness of good postural habits and how to retain them is learned at an early age from the example of adults, so people are often unconscious of whether their posture is good or bad. Most have an image of their posture and stance as it once was, but body alignment can change as we age, often becoming distorted by bad sitting habits or working practices acquired over time. We seldom change our sense and awareness of our body image, however, even if the reflexes become badly affected by bad posture. The inner eye carries an image of posture that is upright and all right. Only in a shop window reflection or through a comment made by another person do we sometimes catch sight of the truth.

Travellers who grew up in countries of the industrialized West, where people commonly suffer from postural defects, often comment on the graceful movements and stance of people from indigenous cultures, who enjoy healthier postural habits.

But their understanding of the body alignment that produces natural grace is often rudimentary, because it is rarely taught in school. Teachers of some sports and fitness regimes try to raise awareness of posture, but are often poorly informed. Postural defects may be seriously discussed only by doctors and physiotherapists when dealing with disorders and illnesses arising from them.

Why slump and slouch?

What causes poor posture? As well as the example of our parents, the things we do as daily routine at home or at work are a major source – slumping in front of the TV; sitting at a computer all day. Some hobbies and professions demand that the body be used in particular ways. For example, ballet dancers walk with turned-out feet, causing the shortening of the outside muscles of the legs. Some people are trained as dancers from early childhood, so the knees and hips may be permanently deformed as a result. Ida Rolf points to even earlier conditioning: the habit of clothing toddlers in thick nappies forces them to develop abnormal walking movements. Later, certain jobs, such as gardening or laying paving, or habitually carrying a baby on one hip, can make the back curve forward or distort the lower spine over time, causing chronic backache.

Cool fashions and body language can train the body into bad habits. Fashionable shoes may look sensational, but they can inhibit the function of the feet. In extreme fashions, such as stiletto-heeled, pointed-toed shoes, the toes are squashed and distorted at the joints.

Dynamic stance

Fitness instruction books often depict good posture by showing a person standing with head erect, seat tucked in, stomach pulled in, and legs and feet parallel. A person in this position is not standing badly, but posture is not static. Almost every part of the body is involved in standing upright, and the correct alignment of all body parts must be maintained when sitting, crouching, kneeling, walking, running, and turning round to see something.

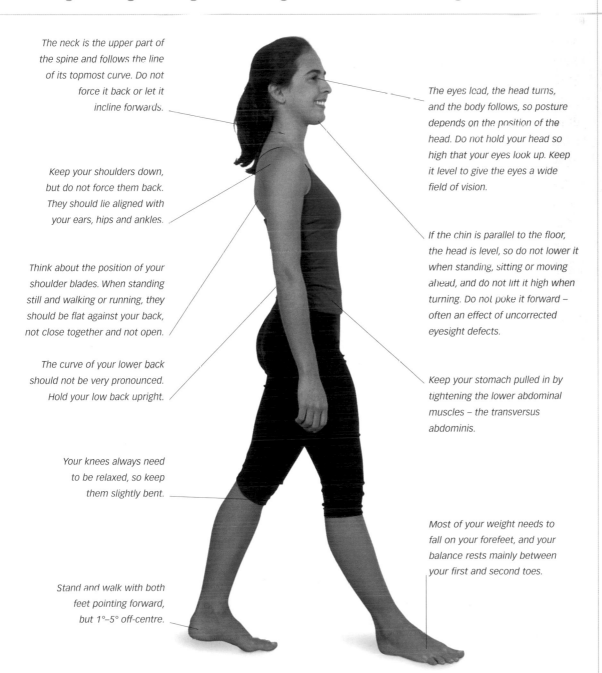

The neck is the upper part of the spine and follows the line of its topmost curve. Do not force it back or let it incline forwards.

Keep your shoulders down, but do not force them back. They should lie aligned with your ears, hips and ankles.

Think about the position of your shoulder blades. When standing still and walking or running, they should be flat against your back, not close together and not open.

The curve of your lower back should not be very pronounced. Hold your low back upright.

Your knees always need to be relaxed, so keep them slightly bent.

Stand and walk with both feet pointing forward, but 1°–5° off-centre.

The eyes lead, the head turns, and the body follows, so posture depends on the position of the head. Do not hold your head so high that your eyes look up. Keep it level to give the eyes a wide field of vision.

If the chin is parallel to the floor, the head is level, so do not lower it when standing, sitting or moving ahead, and do not lift it high when turning. Do not poke it forward – often an effect of uncorrected eyesight defects.

Keep your stomach pulled in by tightening the lower abdominal muscles – the transversus abdominis.

Most of your weight needs to fall on your forefeet, and your balance rests mainly between your first and second toes.

Self-assessment

Every body has unique structural strengths and weaknesses, so everyone has different exercise requirements. One person has lower back pain and needs to improve spinal flexibility; another wants to rehabilitate an injured ankle. Pilates exercises are designed to adapt to people's different requirements. It is essential for your holistic health to know all the key exercises in Part 5, but you will also need to develop a customized exercise plan. An important early step is to assess your body's needs. If you practise pilates without a teacher you must learn to assess your own posture and identify your own priorities.

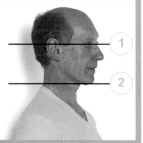

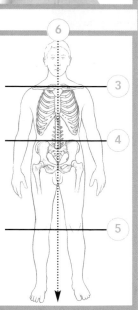

Develop an awareness of your body alignments. To maintain good balance and posture, be aware of the horizontal alignments – the eyes and their sightline (1), the chin (2), the shoulders (3), the hips (4), and the knees (5). They keep the plumbline (6) falling vertically down the midline.

Some exercise systems make everyone repeat the same physical actions, encouraging the development of a particular type of physique and ignoring individual physical makeup. Consequently, even people who have exercised for years may not know their own body. To begin pilates is to embark on a self-assessment that becomes an ongoing exercise in self-awareness, and should last until your body stops changing. Start by examining your body and trying to assess its structural problems, then try to raise your awareness of how you sit in trains, at a desk, while talking on the telephone, when lifting and carrying something heavy. Look out for reflections of your posture in a window or a mirror when you walk through a door, run to catch a lift, wait in a queue, and get out of a car seat.

If you work at a computer, stop now and again and think about the position of your head and shoulders; if you work in catering or another job involving bending over a work surface, check the curve of your upper spine. Dancers should look at the angle of their feet when they walk, and tennis players at the symmetry of their arms and shoulders. Think back: at school, did you carry a heavy bag over one shoulder? This is disastrous for balanced development of left and right sides of the body during the growth spurt. Is your body flexible and coordinated, or does it feel stiff, awkward and clumsy?

Preventing ill health

The answers to some of these questions are likely to point in the direction of future illnesses even if you have no symptoms now. For example, how does stress affect your posture when you are driving or dealing with frustrations at home? Do you let it linger on, unresolved, or do you walk, run, swim or play a sport regularly? Do you flog your body to make it meet your ambitions or your exercise goals? The body's reactions to overwork and injuries often take the form of misalignments of the frame and over- or underuse of certain muscles. These show up as defects in the way we stand or move. Over-vigorous exercise can put the back out, affect the alignment of the knees, or weaken the arches of the feet.

As you work through the exercises in Part 5, those you find hardest often reflect hidden structural defects. For example, if you cannot stand on one leg easily, the psoas muscle may be weak. Once you understand which areas of your body need attention, you can work out which exercise to focus on in your programme.

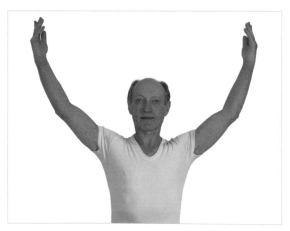

Can you raise your arms above your head, keeping shoulders and lats right down? This means rotating them at the shoulders (see page 47). If not, the joints may be inflamed or the muscles weak. To restructure: practise the arm circles on pages 107–08.

Checking alignments

Study your image in a mirror, or ask someone to photograph you from the front, the back and the side, and examine the photograph carefully, looking for the following points. Placing the photograph on a piece of squared paper makes it easier to see misalignments, whether, for instance, one hip or shoulder is higher than the other, as in this image:

1 *Is your head straight, or tipped to one side? The back of the head should be aligned with the spine and level with the chin. The eyeline should be level.*
To restructure: *Your neck and shoulder muscles may be tight from lack of use or working at a desk. Tight muscles on one side of the neck can cause earache. Massage your neck and work on the exercises on pages 94–95.*

2 *Are your shoulders parallel to the floor – or Is one higher or held further forward than the other?*
To restructure: *Perhaps you carry a shoulder bag – or did you, in the past, carry a school bag over one shoulder? Work on realigning arms and shoulders with the exercises on pages 98–100.*

3 *Are your hip bones parallel to the floor, or is one higher than the other?*
To restructure: *If your hips are misaligned, the quadratus lumborum may be tight and pulling your body over. Practise the Waist stretcher, page 102.*

4 *Do you walk with feet turned out?*
To restructure: *Walking with splayed feet can cause knee, hip and back problems. Walk with your feet pointing forward, but just off-centre, and work on the foot exercises on pages 110–11.*

5 *Is your spine straight when seen from behind? When seen from the side, do its curves seem natural, or is one of them flattened or too pronounced?*
To restructure: *Misalignment of the spine causes backache. The stretch on page 179 will relieve it, then practise the Diving stance on page 112 and the Low back and thigh stretch on page 120.*

6 *Do your shoulder blades stick out?*
To restructure: *Your serratus anterior or rhomboids are tight (see page 49). Practise the back stretch on pages 98–99 and the Cat stretch on page 103.*

7 *Walk and turn in front of a full-length mirror. Does your behind protrude? Do you walk unevenly?*
To restructure: *Your tailbone may be held too high – practise the Head and neck curl on page 96.*

8 *Is one foot inverted – twisted so the sole turns inward? This distorts posture and causes pain in the calf, knee, hip and back.*
To restructure: *Your heel, forefoot and toes must all touch the ground when you take a step, as shown by the triangle (left).*

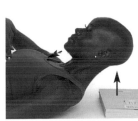

How strong are your neck muscles?

Lie on your back on the floor with your hands by your sides. Without using your arms, try to lift your head until your chin touches your chest. If your neck muscles are weak, you will have to move your head to one side to lift it. Weakened neck muscles cannot support the head, and that causes postural imbalance from head to toe. The neck-strengthening exercises on pages 176–77 help correct this imbalance.

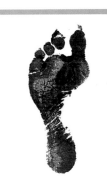

Your footprint tells you whether you have well-structured feet with strongly supported arches, as indicated by the curve in the instep of the foot above. If the curve is poorly defined or absent, your arches may be weak or collapsed. Work on the foot exercises on pages 110–11, and see a chiropodist.

Remodelling

Pilates exercises interact with the body structure to improve alignment and restore impaired function to joints and muscles, creating confidence and a sense of wellbeing. But to fully restructure a neglected and unexercised body, and to rehabilitate it after strain or injury, it is essential to fulfil three conditions. First, you must have a thorough understanding of the condition of your body, its postural defects, and its structural weaknesses, based on a realistic assessment. Second, you need to work toward a set of achievable goals. And third, to achieve your aims you must persevere with the full exercise programme.

Whatever the results of your self-assessment (see pages 64–65), the first stage in restructuring and remodelling the body is to balance it. Your assessment will have revealed imbalances – hunched shoulders, perhaps, or a slightly lopsided walk, which is often the result of uneven development. For example, a person who sits all day at work, then drives home and sits for most of the evening, will tend to have tight hip flexors, hamstrings and calf muscles. These need to be stretched to balance them so that you feel secure against gravity. The exercises on pages 112–21 do this.

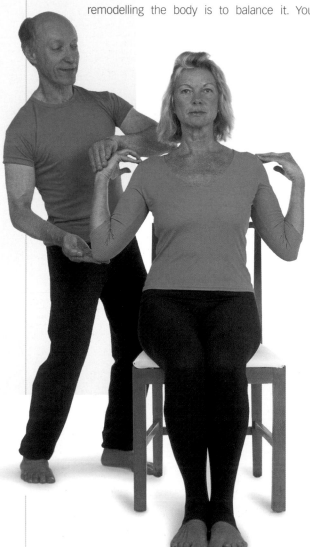

Pilates treats the body holistically, so problems are not remedied by repeating exercises mindlessly. The key exercises in Part 5 (marked with a key symbol) will remedy defects of posture and body structure if practised together as a programme about three times a week. The exercises in Part 5 are progressive – they are divided into levels and stages, but to maintain structural fitness it will always be necessary to include Level 1 exercises in your regular programme. This often comes as a surprise to beginners, who do not expect that in ten years' time they will be working through exercises they learned in the first weeks of practice. They may be essential, however, to flatten a protruding stomach (page 55), ease a frozen shoulder into mobility (page 47), or restore coordination between left and right legs after a knee injury.

No physique is perfect, but every body is improvable and no matter how imperfect you think you look or how rigid you feel, you can change for the better. The body is a pliable structure – the muscles can stretch at any age if they are exercised gently. A qualified pilates teacher can help you decide how best to work on your body to realise your physical potential.

Making progress

Each exercise gives you new information, and as you work through the programme the experience of exercising changes. At the start, certain exercises may seem simple and others more difficult than they should be. The movements that seem hardest may indicate some structural problem that escaped your self-assessment. For example, a person who finds the Lower back and thigh stretch on page 120 hard may be dealing with stiffness in the lumbar part of the spine, although they may have no back pain. Change happens quickly, so by about the sixth practice session the stretch may have become easier. Level 1 exercises (see pages 88–139) go straight to the commonly neglected and structurally unfit areas of the body: the neck and shoulders, the lower back, the abdomen and the feet, revealing weaknesses.

On the other hand, an exercise that you have always found easy can unaccountably start to seem difficult. Everyone has blind spots, and you may have been skimping an essential step or have misunderstood a movement. Mind and body change as you progress, and you may suddenly have got the point of an exercise and started trying to do it properly. Gradually, the whole body responds to the attention given to its separate parts.

Goals to aim for

Structural fitness WILL:

- Improve your posture so you move more gracefully.
- Tone and streamline your body and make you stand tall.
- Make you fit so you have more energy and feel great.
- Keep you flexible and mobile into old age.

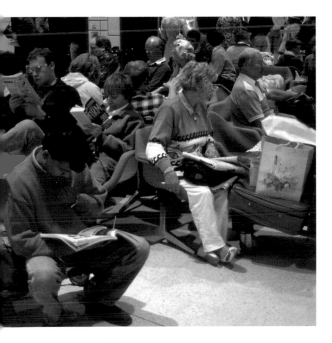

Time will tell how much effort you put into correcting and refining your posture over the years. Wherever you are, whatever you are doing, remind yourself to sit and stand upright with your head up and your shoulders down and open.

Structural fitness will NOT:

- Give you the body of a supermodel if the body you want is structurally different from the one you were born with.
- Give you long, thin legs if your legs are not naturally long and thin.
- Make you lose weight or make you thinner:
  Note: If you are seriously overweight, you need to slim down by combining a healthy diet with gentle daily walking before starting the exercises. A change of eating habits and regular gentle aerobic exercise need to be combined with structural fitness exercises to help you lose weight.

Correcting injuries

Injuries can cause postural defects. A broken bone may mend easily, but regaining use of the limb, hip or shoulder may take longer. You tend to protect the damaged area by underusing it, and this habit can persist after the bone is mended. If physiotherapy fails to counter this imbalance, carry out a self-assessment to see how far the affected area is out of alignment with the other side of the body. To restore balanced function, the faulty habit must be replaced by one that works the area in the normal way. Level 1 exercises will stretch and tone the muscles in the affected area, and Level 2 and 3 exercises will strengthen them and integrate their movements into those of your whole body.

Principles of practice

Exercising the pilates way is a skill: you learn a new set of movements and practise them until you can perform them with confidence in a balanced, rhythmic way. To be able to do this involves exercising according to a set of principles and bringing certain qualities into the movements. That involves a clear understanding of exercise, its benefits, and its effects on the body. These pages explain the five basic principles or watchwords of the pilates system, and additional ones that apply to structural fitness. Basing each exercise on these principles and qualities ensures that it will have the desired effect on the body.

1 Breathing

The exercises begin and end with breathing. Mainly under nervous control, but partly controlled by the will, breathing is the link between mind and body. Level 1 exercises encourage breathing using all of the lungs, which speeds the circulation, raises energy levels, and improves concentration and mental functioning. The movements of the diaphragm (the major muscle involved in breathing), the internal muscles of the pelvis (called the pelvic floor, location of the body's centre), and the external abdominal muscles are all interrelated, so breathing can be influenced and changed by the way we use these muscles. Since the pelvic floor muscles play an essential role in maintaining stability, breathing, balance and body control are closely connected. Breath control is therefore an important element in every exercise. Long, slow out-breaths are encouraged in Level 1 exercises; while those in Level 2 teach the control of in-breaths. An in-breath is a preparation for starting a movement, while an out-breath accompanies each movement.

2 Isolation and integration

Pilates exercises restructure and rehabilitate by first isolating the body part or parts affected by imbalance, then by integrating the movements of that body area into the smooth functioning of the whole. They do this by working first on one side of the body and then on the other, stretching the left hip, then the right, exercising the psoas muscle on the right side, then on the left, so that

as you work on each body part, its movement is balanced by exercising its partner on the opposite side. Key integrating exercises occur at intervals through Part 5. These integrating exercises work several major muscle groups at once, coordinating the movements and integrating them into the movements of the whole body.

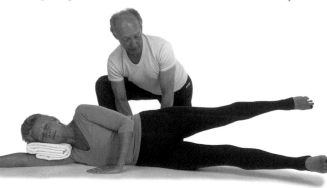

Scissors on pages 186–87 is a key integrating exercise. It works both sides of the body at the same time, coordinating and integrating the actions of the groups of muscles that work the hips and the legs.

3 Precision

The angle of the pelvis, the precise positioning of a foot, even the direction of the gaze are essential to the effectiveness of pilates exercises. The senses must be fully involved in every movement. Precision comes only with practice. If at first an exercise seems not to work, reread the instructions carefully. All through Part 5, the introductions to the exercises, closeups of details, and 'Points to watch' boxes pinpoint important details that make all the difference.

4 Concentration

'Quality, not quantity' is one of the founding principles of pilates. The importance of carrying out exercises with care and deliberation is stressed in the writings of Joseph Pilates, who dismissed exercising on the basis of rapid repetitions. To be effective, pilates exercises need to be done slowly, with the concentration focused on the precision and smooth flow of each movement, and on the goal of the exercise. This may take time to achieve, but it also requires the right conditions. That is why it is important to set aside regular times for practice, and, if possible, to exercise in a quiet room with distractions eliminated. This can be hard for anyone learning at home, but with perseverance and determination it is achievable.

Joseph Pilates might have been horrified by the treadmills and stationary cycling machines in modern gyms, where people move mechanically, their minds paying scant attention to the actions their bodies are making, their sight, hearing and touch scarcely involved in the movements of the muscles. One imagines that he would have improved the quality of the exercise by modifying the use of the apparatus

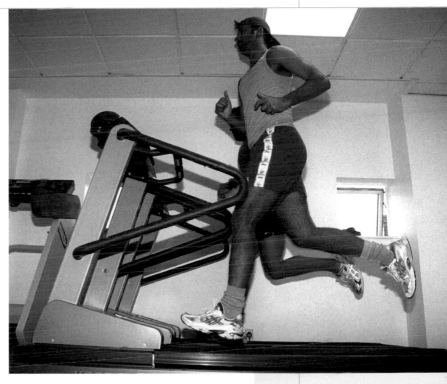

Many sports involve training on gym apparatus, and the British cricketers in the photograph above are working out on treadmills. Like all exercise, gym workouts need to be done with concentration if you are to benefit from them.

5 Control

Exercises carried out smoothly and rhythmically look beautiful because they reflect perfect physical and mental control. This can take years to achieve, but the effort is itself rewarding. Try to stand on one leg for one full minute, and at first you wobble and fall every few seconds. After a week, the wobble is reduced to a waver and you can stand for a full minute. Some months later and you can stand rock-still for as long as you like because you have toned, balanced, strengthened, and you are using all the muscles involved. You can also focus mind and body unwaveringly on accomplishing the task. To gain control involves the whole mind and body. As you practise pilates, the effect of each exercise changes. Each time you repeat one, you learn something new.

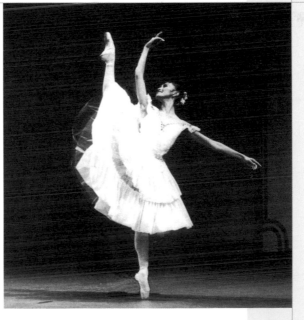

Ballet dancers have to demonstrate perfect control over the balance of the body. Balancing in this position demands full concentration.

6 Centering

To be centered is to be able to maintain good posture and balance no matter what the position of your body or where your legs and arms may be. Centering depends on good control of the muscles of the pelvic floor and an awareness of the body's centre or midpoint. Dancers, skaters and gymnasts are always aware of their centre. As they move and turn, they work around it but never seek to rest on it, for its position changes. Bend your knees and you move it closer to the ground. The Stage 2 exercises make you aware of your centre by teaching you to activate the hidden muscles of the pelvic floor and lift them towards your midpoint. This can be difficult at first, but if you persevere you find that your posture, stability, balance and control radically improve. And because body and mind work in tandem, healthier pelvic floor muscles bring a sense of wellbeing.

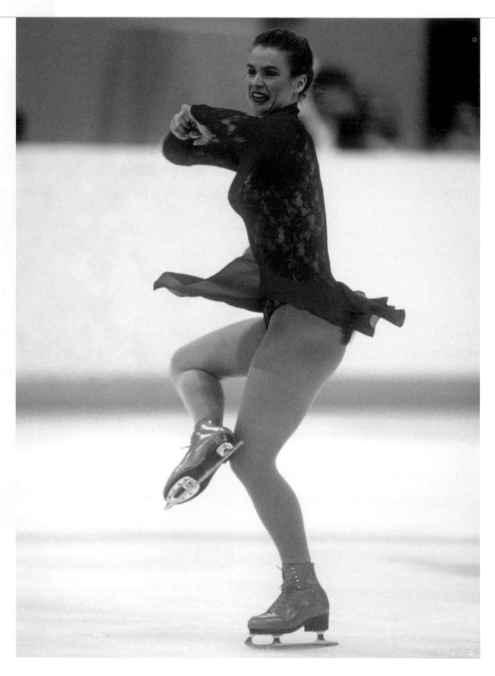

The body's centre or midpoint is the focus of dynamic movement. When skaters, gymnasts or dancers have a bad day and are dissatisfied with their balance, leaps and turns, they often complain that they cannot find their centre.

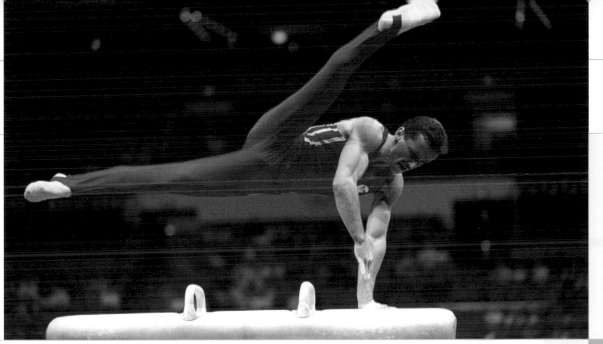

Practice makes perfect because feedback from the proprioceptors (sense receptors in the tissues that inform the brain about the body's position in space) enable mind, nerves, and muscles to work together to achieve core stability and perfect coordination.

7 Balance

When the body's weight is equally and correctly distributed, you can function most efficiently under the additional weight of gravity. Pilates exercises work on perfecting physical balance, and because balance is inextricably associated with mental and emotional equilibrium, they produce mental harmony. Balancing the muscles in pilates exercises corrects one-sided and uncoordinated muscle action. If muscle fibres are unused, they shorten, causing the muscle to tighten. The exercises stretch them and make them contract. They exercises also work muscles that operate together as agonists and antagonists (see page 45) to coordinate their actions. And bilateral muscles (on both sides of the body) are exercised separately and together to integrate the movements of the left and right sides. Each exercise serves as yardstick and measure for the muscles involved. Are they taut, are they too slack? How are they affecting posture? These are questions you need to ask as part of your self-assessment (see pages 64–65)

8 Flowing movement

It is impossible at the beginning not to stop moving while thinking out where a foot should be placed, and not to hasten over a familiar movement. Only when you know the movements thoroughly can you think about rhythm and flow. Their pace and rhythm are set by the out-breath. From the start of the exercises in Part 5 you learn to move while breathing out slowly to a rhythmic count of six. Flow comes

from exercising each part of the body to its full potential, the limbs stretched out while describing their circles and half-circles evenly; lifting from the centre and extending the lift into a stretch up the spine to the top of the head. Flow comes from learning not to jerk at the changeover from lifting or lowering to arching or circling; never moving too fast, speeding up, or slowing down; and maintaining a rhythmic count while stretching, holding a stretch, and relaxing at the end of it.

9 Relaxation

Tension and stress influence health. They undermine the balance of the body by tightening muscles and restricting the breathing, preventing spontaneous movement. The muscles tighten and the breathing speeds up in response to a sudden alarm. If the tension is not dispelled, they fail to relax again afterwards, and this is how stress becomes chronic. The exercise programme begins on page 84–85 with self-massage. This is not included in most pilates programmes, yet not only does it ease tight muscles but it can also help remove one of the causes of tension, for some people experience stress when exercising or focusing on the body. Massaging yourself is a good way for a beginner to learn relaxation. It puts you in contact with who you are.

A graceful exercising style is a core quality of pilates and something to aim for. The special midpoint lift (see page 137) will help you attain flowing movement.

Many exercise systems end with a short relaxation session like the one on pages 204–05. It makes a useful transition between exercising and going back to the outside world, and it is an excellent way to prepare for sleep.

Aerobic vs. structural fitness

People who have never exercised the pilates way often begin by working through the exercises as if they are trying to break a world sprinting record. They approach pilates as if it were aerobics. The exercises should be done neither at speed nor so slowly that the muscles scarcely know where a movement begins and ends, but at a measured, rhythmic pace. In fact, the body also needs aerobic exercise, because it increases the amount of oxygen in the blood and strengthens the heart and the lungs, whereas pilates exercises build overall strength, endurance and flexibility. The two are different, but compatible, and these pages show how they may be combined.

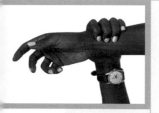

Find your resting pulse rate by taking your pulse after sitting reading for ten minutes, then compare the result with the rate after exercising.

With any effort that raises the body's temperature, the pulse rate is equal to the number of beats the heart has to make to pump oxygen-rich blood from the lungs around the body quickly enough to maintain normal functioning, and so restore normal temperature. The more unfit the body, the harder the heart has to work, and the higher the pulse rate. The pulse is therefore used as an indicator of the condition of the heart, the lungs, and the muscles. It is also a measure of emotional stress.

The resting pulse rate of a fit person is around 72 beats per minute for men, 75 for women, 80 for boys, and 84 for girls, with individual variations. A rate of over 80 for an adult at rest indicates that the heart is pumping faster than normal. During exercise, the muscles under our voluntary control normally contract strongly, then release, and this rhythmic action squeezes the underlying veins. In the legs, this helps pump the blood up to the heart. If the muscles are flabby, however, their action on the veins is reduced and has to be made up by the heart working harder than it should. Since the heart is a muscle, the tone and coordinated action of its fibres are weakened, increasing the strain on its pumping action. Any extra effort is reflected in a heightened pulse rate.

Achieving aerobic fitness

To regain fitness the resting heart rate must be lowered, for this, the quality of the heart muscle and the actions of its fibres need to become more coordinated. This can be achieved through short periods of exertion which raise the heartbeat and exercise the heart, strengthening its tone and pumping action. In time, the strengthened heart beats far more effectively, so that when the body rests after exercise the heart returns to its resting beat more quickly, and fewer beats per minute are needed to service it. The resting pulse rate is therefore reduced.

Aerobic activities that exercise the heart and reduce the resting pulse rate include brisk walking, jogging, running, cycling, swimming and aerobic dance. To achieve a reasonable standard of fitness, you need to carry out one of these activities for 10 to 20 minutes a session, three times a week, reading your pulse before and after each session. If you do not know how to read your pulse, it is explained simply in all first aid books.

Resting heart rate

For any activity to be aerobically effective, you target a heart rate of between 55% and 90% of your maximum heart rate, which is 220 beats a minute minus your age. From now on, check your pulse rate at the end of every session of aerobic activity and aim to achieve a rate equal to 55–90% of that maximum rate.

> **220** [maximum heart rate in beats per minute]
>
> − **35** [minus your age]
>
> = **185** beats per minute

Aim at a rate of 101–166 beats per minute.

The exercise ball

A very safe and gentle way of working the heart and lungs is to bounce on an exercise ball – the ball takes the strain instead of the body. Also called 'medicine balls', they are available from exercise stores and can be used safely by people of all ages. They do not take up much space, so they may be kept at home and they are popular with children. You can begin a structural fitness session with the exercises on this page, or do them separately at any other time. Bouncing is the aerobic activity in the first part of the exercise, but the second part is structural – you can only do it if you lift the internal muscles of the pelvis (called the pelvic floor, see pages 129–34).

1 Begin by sitting on the ball to get the feel of it, and gently bounce up and down. When you are confident, try turning to the left and the right while continuing to bounce, keeping your feet pressing down on the floor.

2 Sit on the ball and bounce up and down. Lift one foot off the floor and stretch your arms out sideways, then raise them above your head. Repeat, lifting the other foot.

Warning

Do not attempt aerobic exercise before having a medical checkup. Aerobic exercise of any kind can be dangerous if you suffer from angina pectoralis or other heart-related illnesses.

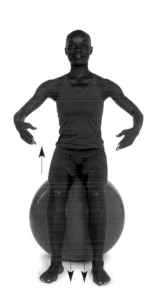
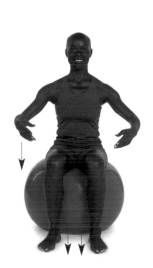
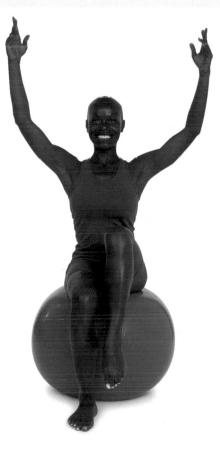

Avoiding impact injuries

The problem with aerobic exercise is that it strains the body. To reach the speed needed to increase the heart rate significantly, the activity has to be repeated at an intensity and for a duration that together cause heavy breathing, sweating and shaking. The body temperature is normally 37° C (98.6° F), but during fast aerobic exercise it rises towards 40° C (100° F). As it rises, the lungs and heart have to work at well above normal speed to supply enough oxygen and glucose for the muscles to work so hard and the body to maintain its systems.

The moment the action stops, the body restores the stable internal environment it needs to regulate the body systems. Resting returns the heart and breathing rates to normal. Fluid lost by sweating to lower the temperature can be replaced by drinking water. In time, the heart strengthens and pumps more blood more quickly; and lung capacity expands so that more oxygen can be taken in with each breath.

The effects of aerobic exercise are now so well known that physical fitness is equated by many people with aerobic fitness. But since the 1970s craze for aerobic exercise, the exercising public has also become aware of its downside: it puts strain on the heart, and in an unfit person this might result in a heart attack. Moreover, during jogging, running or jumping, all the body weight is transferred to one leg each time the heel hits the ground. Studies of five marathon runners found that a force of more than two and a half times the weight of the body is loaded on to one leg, knee, ankle and foot with each step. Forces of 3.6 times body weight have been recorded during sprinting. Body structures cannot always stand up to such a pounding, which jars the joints, damaging the knees, hips and spine, and can cause impact fractures.

There are easier ways of achieving aerobic fitness. In addition to the exercise ball (see page 73), an effective way of achieving aerobic fitness without causing structural damage is to use a trampoline or a bouncer (mini-trampoline). These may be ordered from sports equipment suppliers and can be used safely at all ages.

They do not take up much space, so they may be kept at home. Most children also love playing on them. You can begin a structural fitness session with aerobic exercises on this equipment.

Trampolines and bouncers

A beginner can achieve aerobic fitness quickly by progressing from bouncing continuously for a minute or two at first, to 5 minutes or more after a session or two, and eventually to 15 minutes. Bouncing can be especially helpful for anyone who cannot walk far or is recovering from an ankle or knee injury, since the downward impact of the body weight on the joints is reduced to a minimum. The energy used by the muscles on every rebound is reduced, so many more repetitions can be attempted before the muscles get tired and their performance quality is affected. In time, bouncing improves the body's proprioceptive responses (see page 34) so that the time it takes to adjust to new positions is reduced. Bouncing is also a good way of restoring the body's metabolism and getting the circulation and breathing going.

Points to watch

- Be sure the bouncer is properly set up according to the maker's instructions, and is safe for bouncing before you step on it.

- Always use a support. At first, use a support bar. When you feel more confident, lean with your hands against a wall for support during the rebound to maintain control and balance.

- To increase the breathing rate and encourage deep breathing, try to breathe out on an even count of six.

- When you finish, step off the bouncer. Never bounce, then jump from the bouncer down to the floor. This can seriously impact the joints and the lower back.

Learning to bounce

Begin by reading your resting pulse rate (see page 72) so you can check how quickly it responds and improves. Start by stepping gently onto the trampoline or bouncer and practise bouncing up and down slowly. It is the rebound from the feet that moves the body up and down, so your knees must be very slightly bent all the time. Do not bend them too much or you will deaden the rebound and come to a jerky halt. When you feel confident, attempt the following exercise. Start slowly, and speed up as you become more confident.

1 Step carefully onto the bouncer, stand with both feet together, and bend your knees slightly. Practise moving up and down. Once you are bouncing to a rhythm, start lifting up and replacing each knee in turn while continuing to bounce to the same rhythm.

2 After bouncing to a rhythm for a while, try jumping, lifting both knees together during the bounce up.

3 When you have practised for a while, try jumping higher, then do five high jumps in succession.

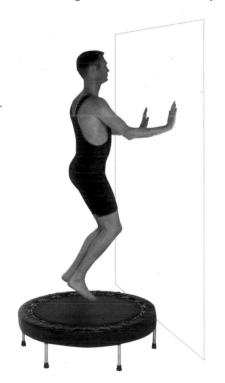 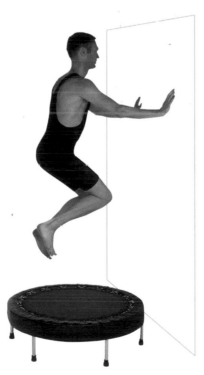 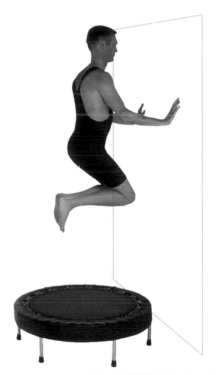

Finish and rest

When you have finished bouncing, step carefully off the bouncer and do the Lower back and thigh stretch (see page 120) or, if you can, the Bear stretch (see page 121) to lengthen the hamstrings and stretch the lower back. Then rest.

variation

- Bounce up and down four times on both feet, then on alternating feet, then try to jump high from the left foot, then the right, left again, then right. Repeat.
- Now speed up so that you are running. When you are used to this, try to run for 20 long out-breaths.

part 5
the exercises

Before any real benefit can be derived from
physical exercises, one must first learn how to
breathe properly. Our very life depends on it.

JOSEPH PILATES

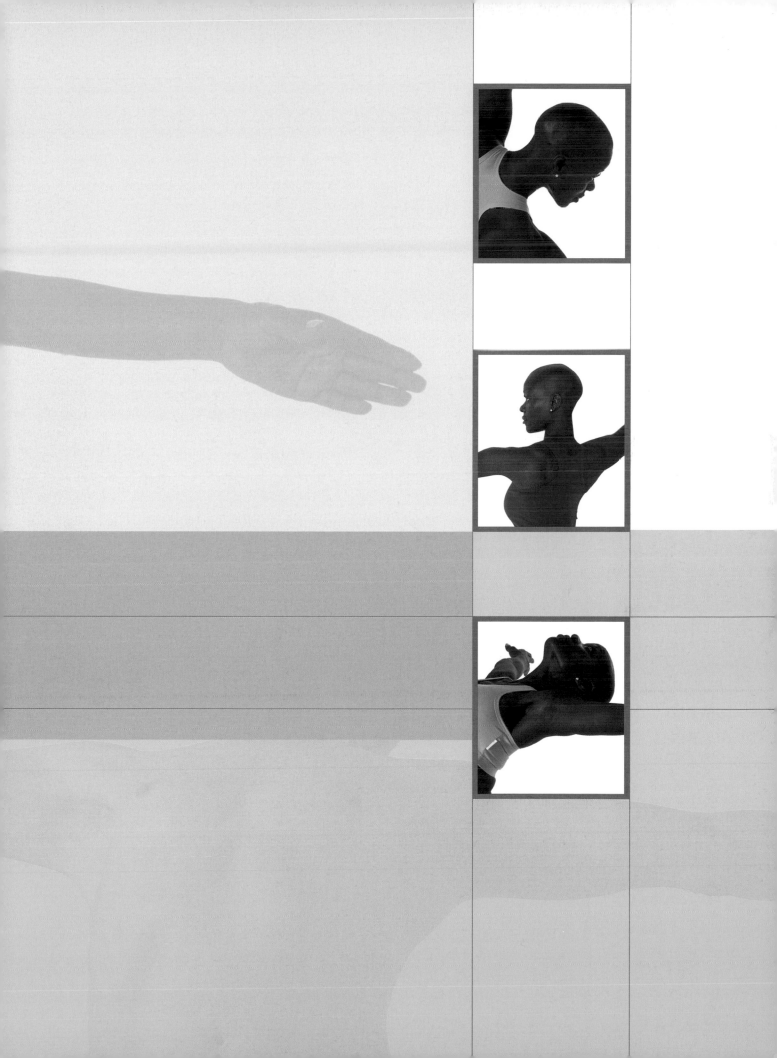

Approaching exercise

Now you have read all about my exercise method and learned how your body moves and how your muscles work, it is time to begin exercising. This chapter presents a full programme of exercises for you to work through. If you are a beginner, work through at your own pace, but expect to take at least 12 weeks to learn all the exercises in this chapter. By the end of the twelfth week, all your skeletal muscles will be stretched, their tone will be improved, and they will be stronger. You will have better posture and your movements will be more coordinated.

I always start my sessions with therapeutic massage, and you should do the same. This is not a pilates technique, but one of my own, inspired by the Swedish pioneer of structural fitness, Per Henrik Ling (see page 17). People who neglect exercise or whose exercise consists mainly of sports such as tennis or golf that work one side of the body more than the other, are often uncoordinated. Some muscles are overused and some underused. I find that massage helps my clients work towards a balance by easing rigidities created by tension. For example, the shoulder blades may be unnaturally high because the rhomboids and the lats are over-tight and unable to pull them back. Massage helps relax and free these muscles.

Remember that balance is one of the principles of structural fitness (see page 71). We speak of 'the psoas' or 'the vastus medialis' as if the body had only one of each, but our bodies are bilateral (two-sided) and most muscles occur on both sides: there is a psoas on the left and one on the right. For this reason, you need to carry out most exercises first on one side, then on the other.

Levels and stages

The programme is broken up into three levels. Since effective exercising depends on controlled breathing, each level begins with breathing exercises, which are a good way of warming up. Level 1 concentrates mainly on the upper body and it works at correcting posture. I start with the upper body, because the placement of the head and neck indicates the balance of the body posture (see page 35). Level 1 has two stages: Stage 1 stretches the muscles of the trunk, extends the spine, opens the

shoulder girdle and the hips, works the legs, and rotates the feet. Stage 2 focuses on exercising the pelvic floor.

Many women learn pelvic floor exercises at antenatal classes because the importance of the pelvic floor's role in pregnancy and childbirth is recognized. However, most people are unaware that it also has a pivotal function in maintaining posture and balance. Women are rarely taught that keeping the pelvic floor fit becomes almost more important in later life than during pregnancy. And few men realize that it is as essential for them to exercise the pelvic floor as it is for women. Level 1 raises awareness of how this hidden part of the body contributes to fitness, and teaches how and when to exercise and lift the pelvic floor.

Level 1 enables you to analyze your body. For example, the Shoulder roll on page 91 indicates how flexible or rigid your shoulders are. These and many other exercises are carried out against a wall. It is easy to see how much closer to the wall you can get a shoulder or a hip or a heel today than you could last week, so the wall helps you measure your progress.

Level 2 and 3 exercises tone and strengthen the muscles of the lower body particularly, and improve coordination and integration. For these more advanced exercises you move away from the wall and get acquainted with the floor. Deprived of the wall's support, you find the exercises more difficult. Level 3 ends with a few minutes of total relaxation, giving time for stretched muscles to rest. When you know all the exercises up to the end of Level 3, I hope that regular structural fitness exercises will be part of your daily life.

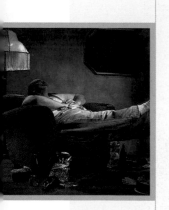

Relaxation in front of the TV – or training in poor posture? Riding to work, sitting all day, riding back, and slumping on a sofa all add up to immobility. If immobility becomes a habit, it can encourage blood clots to form in the deep leg veins, which may lead to a stroke.

Key symbol

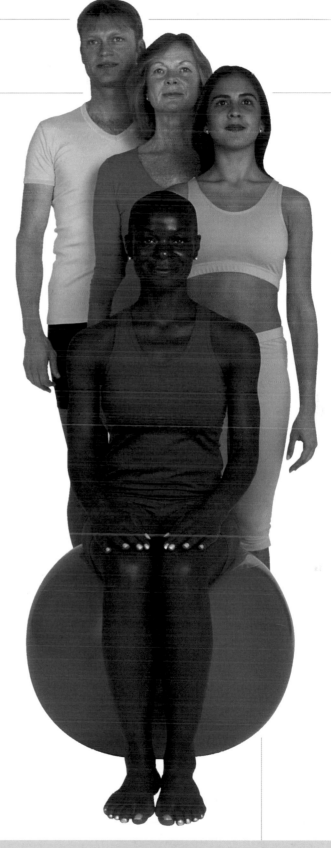

This symbol identifies key exercises at all three levels. Once you have worked through the exercises on pages 88–203, you will need to focus on these key exercises to maintain structural fitness. Pages 80–83 give guidelines for planning a fitness maintenance program based on the key exercises.

Guidelines

- The exercises are progressive and should be done in the order shown in this chapter.
- Plan to practise for about an hour at a time every two or three days.
- Do not try to get through too much in one session. Work through the programme at your own speed, focusing on one or two exercises in a session.
- Do each exercise slowly. Good results come only from concentrating on the movements and how the body feels.
- Before trying a new exercise, read through the instructions and get a mental picture of how to do it. Rest afterwards, then reread and try again.
- Always relax between repetitions to allow the muscles to rest after stretching. End each session with the relaxation exercise on pages 204–05.
- Once you have worked through all the exercises, continue practising for an hour a day three times a week to keep your fitness level high.

People are rarely trained in good habits of posture, movement, and exercise. Many of us have such a sedentary lifestyle that the body is not given the minimum of exertion it needs to be fit and healthy.

As a lifelong avoider of all unnecessary exercise, I came reluctantly to Dreas; but his lucidity and persuasiveness soon converted me. The results include considerable improvements in my stamina, height, and sense of well-being. CHRISTOPHER HAMPTON, PLAYWRIGHT, TRANSLATOR, AND FILM DIRECTOR

Planning your programme

As you work through the exercises in Part 5 and gain confidence with pilates training, you should find you learn more about your body and its needs. When you have reached the end of Level 3, it will be time to review your structural fitness requirements and plan a programme suited to your lifestyle. Like many people, you may want to follow a weekly programme that enables you to maintain the level of structural fitness you have achieved. Alternatively, you may want to work on a particular structural weakness; or, if you run or play a high-impact sport, you may want a few exercises to do before you begin or after you finish in order to avoid structural damage. These pages give you some guidelines to follow.

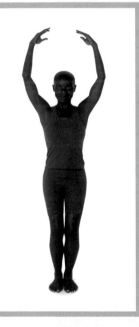

Simple movements take practice. This demonstrator has perfectly positioned and aligned her head, shoulders, hips, knees, ankles, heels and feet, so her body is working in total harmony.

People learn at different speeds and some exercises take longer to learn than others. If you progress more slowly than you expected, bear in mind that your body benefits as you learn each new exercise. If you practise regularly, you speed up, because your mind and body become more attuned to the movements.

When you reach the end of Level 3, your body and its exercise requirements will have changed. Some imbalances and aspects of posture will have improved, and you should notice structural defects that escaped you before. For example, any tension you noticed in your upper back should have eased, but you may become aware of poor flexibility in your hips or lower back.

Fitness maintenance

Of the 85 or more structural fitness exercises in Part 5, many are merely steps that enable you to learn a number of key exercises. These are marked with a key symbol:

They are exercises you should focus on in your personal fitness programme.

Think about maintaining a balance when selecting exercises for your programme. Without a teacher's advice, you must discipline yourself not to fall back on your favourite stretches and avoid other exercises. People often enjoy stretching their arms out against the wall (see pages 98–101), but tend to skip the Shoulder roll

on page 94, perhaps because they find it difficult. It may be tempting to concentrate on the waist, hips, and thighs, but you also need to think holistically and include exercises that stretch and tone the neck and upper body, the lower back, the pelvic floor, and the legs, feet and arms. This allows scope for including extra hip, thigh sand waist stretches, plus a favourite or two.

Although you move away from Level 1, do not think of leaving it behind. Level 1 exercises are the foundation of fitness maintenance. A good plan could be to devote each of your three weekly sessions to reviewing Level 1, Level 2, and Level 3, in turn. You will exercise all parts of the body, and by revisiting key exercises learned at an earlier stage you continue to become aware of new things about its structure

You and your body change constantly, so you should review your requirements every six months.

Learning session	
While learning, it is a good idea to divide your hour like this:	
1 Massage	5–10 minutes
2 Practise exercises already learned	15–20 minutes
3 Learn new exercises	
(allow 5–15 minutes to learn one)	30 minutes
4 Relaxation	5–10 minutes
Total	**about 1 hour**

Fitness maintenance programme

The next two pages show an example of a balanced exercise session lasting a little over an hour, which will maintain overall fitness if repeated three times a week. The estimated time for each exercise is about 3 minutes. If you take longer, break the session and do half on day 1 and the other half on day 2. If you want to begin or end with massage once a week, or finish with relaxation, add 5–10 minutes.

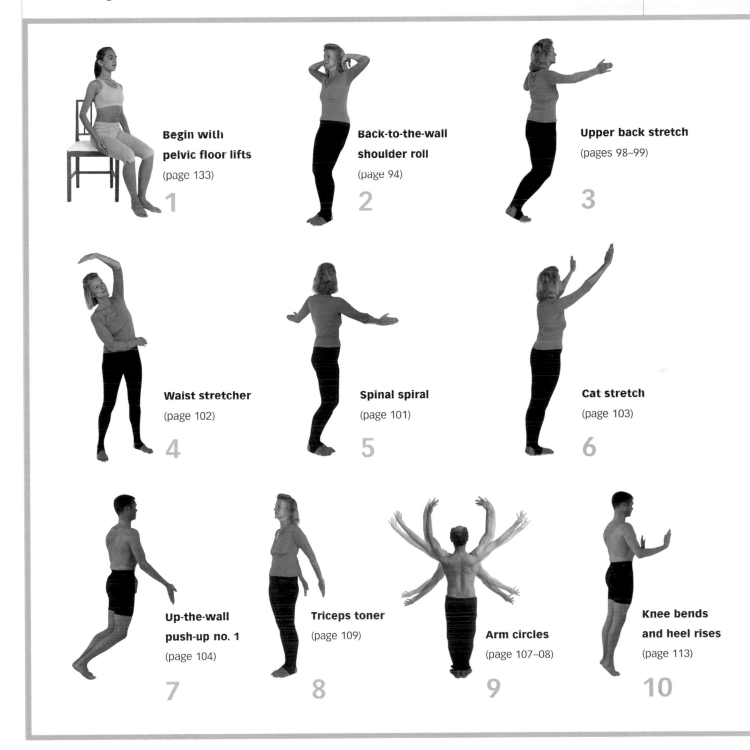

Begin with pelvic floor lifts
(page 133)

1

Back-to-the-wall shoulder roll
(page 94)

2

Upper back stretch
(pages 98–99)

3

Waist stretcher
(page 102)

4

Spinal spiral
(page 101)

5

Cat stretch
(page 103)

6

Up-the-wall push-up no. 1
(page 104)

7

Triceps toner
(page 109)

8

Arm circles
(page 107–08)

9

Knee bends and heel rises
(page 113)

10

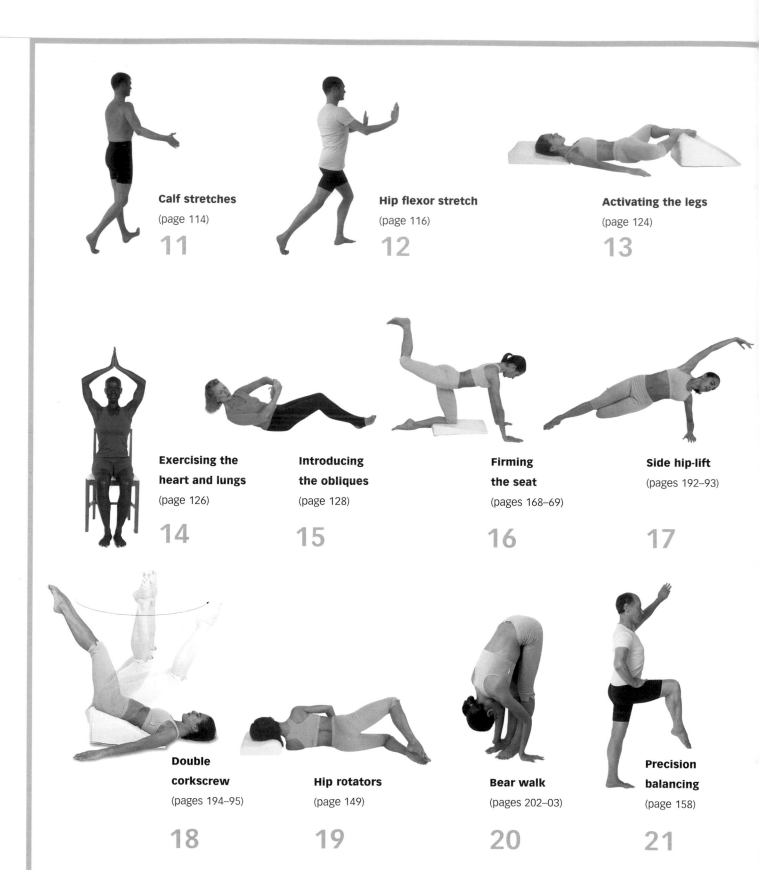

Calf stretches

(page 114)

11

Hip flexor stretch

(page 116)

12

Activating the legs

(page 124)

13

Exercising the heart and lungs

(page 126)

14

Introducing the obliques

(page 128)

15

Firming the seat

(pages 168–69)

16

Side hip-lift

(pages 192–93)

17

Double corkscrew

(pages 194–95)

18

Hip rotators

(page 149)

19

Bear walk

(pages 202–03)

20

Precision balancing

(page 158)

21

Special programmes for special situations – workday programme

Some exercises involve minimal movement so you can practise them anywhere – during a break from the computer, or while waiting for a precooked meal to heat up. Here is a short sequence of exercises for anyone who does a sedentary job. Pushing down with the feet and lifting the pelvic floor are movements that are unlikely to be noticed by other people, so you can take a short break from work now and again and do them at your desk.

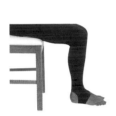 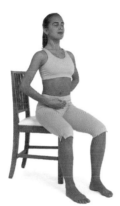 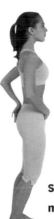 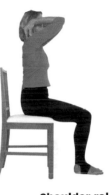

Stabilizing down-push (page 90)

1

Slow pelvic floor lift (page 133)

2

Special midpoint lift (page 137)

3

Shoulder roll (page 91)

4

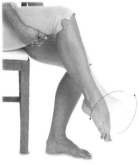 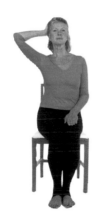 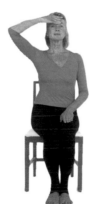 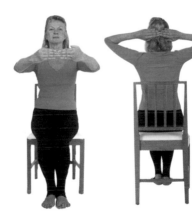

Foot rotations (page 110)

5

Neck strengtheners (page 175)

6

Starting with massage

Massage plus frequent and regular exercise sessions makes the best combination of techniques for improving body posture rapidly. For a beginner, massage is especially useful to correct rigidity in the neck and upper back. The hands can stretch and ease tight shoulder muscles. Balancing exercises then establish new patterns of posture and movement, erasing the imprinting of earlier, structurally incorrect ones. It is expensive and sometimes inconvenient to arrange to be massaged by a professional, but self-massage can be surprisingly effective. These pages introduce ways of massaging the soft tissues using the hands, plus some unorthodox massage aids.

Through years of experience in correcting postural imbalances, I have learned to begin each person's programme with massage. An essential first step is to release the serratus anterior muscles to free the muscles that move the shoulder blades (see page 49). Mental tension is commonly expressed in rigidity of the upper body, and many people arrive with the symptoms: the shoulders dropped forwards, the shoulder blades fixed to the ribs, the head tilted back, the chin lifted, and the neck stiff. The middle spine may curve, making the upper body look hunched.

Touching the sides of the neck often reveals how one-sided a body can be. We get tension headaches and are surprised at the tightness and pain we feel when we touch the muscles. These symptoms gradually disappear as full circulation is restored, first to the muscles, then to the head. Applied at the beginning of a practice session, massage equalizes muscle tone on both sides of the body. The first exercises for the arms and shoulders are consequently more balanced, since equal effort is applied on both sides. Massaging the shoulders relieves tension in the neck and upper spine, so the skull sits more squarely on its pivots: the atlas and axis vertebrae in the neck.

I encourage everyone to begin pilates by massaging these areas three times a week for at least 20 minutes, and then to begin each practice with a short session of 10–12 minutes. Massage can relieve tension all over the body. The feet, always in use but often neglected, respond. These four pages present self-help techniques for massaging the whole body from head to toe. They can all be done wearing a T-shirt or a tracksuit.

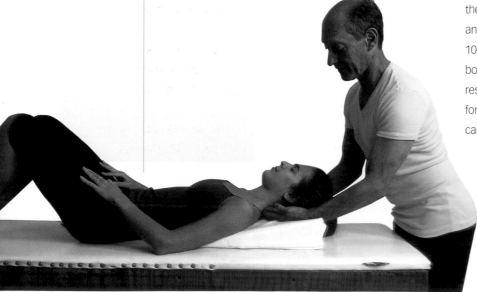

Supplement self-massage with a weekly professional massage. It will help you release rigid muscles more quickly, so they move more freely during exercise sessions. For the first few weeks, while you are working through Level 1, the massage needs to focus on the upper body: the neck, the shoulders and the upper back.

Using the hands

Sit in an upright chair to massage yourself, with your feet on the floor. Begin massaging with either hand, but if your fingers tire at any point change hands and massage the other side of the body, then change back again later. Spend about a minute on each step.

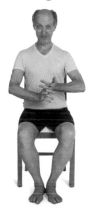 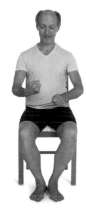 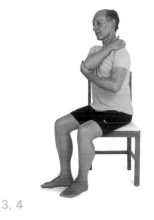 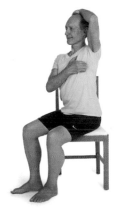

1   2   3, 4   5–7

1 Warm your hands: interlace your fingers and rub the palms together. Unlock the fingers and lace them again, moving one slot along, then massage your palms again.

2 Unlock your fingers, make fists of your hands, then release. Form fists again and circle them from the wrists, clockwise and anticlockwise. Use one hand to stretch the fingers and palm of the opposite hand backwards.

3 Put your right hand on your left shoulder, support the right elbow with your left hand, and search gently for sore spots with your right-hand fingertips along the top of the shoulder blade. Massage them firmly with a circular motion.

4 Move the hand to the ridge between your neck and shoulder, and massage down the upper arm, pressing down with fingers and thumb to find tense spots.

5 Move your left hand up the side of your neck to the top of your skull, then press your fingers down and massage firmly downwards while turning your head slowly from left to right.

6 Rest the fingers of your right hand beside your left shoulder just below the collarbone, and gently massage the muscles of the upper chest towards the breastbone.

7 Place your right-hand fingertips below your left armpit. If the thin serratus anterior muscle beneath them is stretched tightly across your ribs, the rhomboids and trapezius cannot pull your shoulder blades downwards and towards the spine. Massage it to release your shoulder blades.

8 Lift your left elbow and massage gently along and across the ribs with your right hand. The serratus anterior beneath the skin is sensitive, but persevere.

9 Move your right hand up the left side of the neck to the top of your skull and massage very strongly downward, as in step 5.

10 Repeat steps 2–9, crossing the left hand over to the right shoulder and using the left fingers to massage, while supporting the left elbow with the right hand.

Stick massage

A smooth stick about 0.9 metres (3 feet) long is an unorthodox but useful aid to massage, especially for parts of the body the hands cannot reach. Do not use it to massage bony areas, such as the knees or the spine. Stick massage works well over thin clothing because the stick slides over the fabric and does not catch the skin. Grip the stick firmly with both hands and drag it towards the heart. This benefits the circulation. It may be hard at first to drag it upwards while pressing down on it, but it becomes easier with practice.

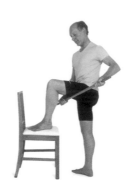

1 **Hamstrings**: stand upright with one foot raised on a chair. Grip the stick with both hands, place it in the fold at the back of the knee, then massage upward with slow strokes. To massage the adductors, work from the back of the knee along the inside of the thigh towards the pelvis.

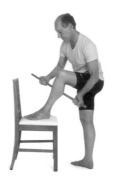

2 **Calf muscles**: Stand upright with one foot resting on a low box or a chair seat, grip the stick with both hands and place it on the ankle, then, pressing it firmly onto the leg, draw it upwards along the calf muscles as shown above. After a few minutes, change feet to massage the other leg.

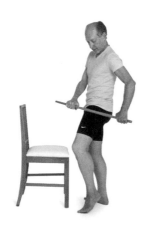

3 **The thigh**: use long upward strokes to massage the iliotibial tract (see page 56), and loosen it after prolonged sitting. Now move the stick to the front of the thigh and, using short, slow upward strokes, work gradually around to the side.

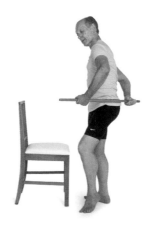

4 **The buttock and above the hip bone**: holding the stick in your right hand, move it behind your body, grasp it with the other hand, and press it against the top of the thigh. Using long, firm strokes, massage upwards to the waist.

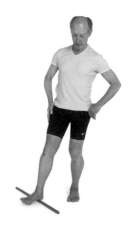

5 **The feet**: put the stick on the floor, place one foot on it and roll the soles and sides of the foot over it, pressing down on any tender spots, then change feet. Sit and rub the stick inside the arches. Massage the upper surface of each foot with the hands.

Tennis ball massage

Tennis balls are an unusual but effective self-help device for massaging the hips, buttocks and muscles of the lower back. Tennis ball massage can be more effective than hand massage for hard-to-reach areas such as an aching upper back or a twinging hip or buttock, since it is easy to regulate your movements. The technique is not difficult, is excellent for massaging the large muscles of the pelvis, and takes little practice.

1 Lie on a mat on your back with your knees bent and feet flat on the floor. Raise your hips, roll the ball beneath your left buttock, and rest your weight on it. Turning slightly towards your left side, use your right foot to move your seat over the ball, massaging your left buttock muscles by moving in small circles over the ball. Keep the ball beneath the soft tissues of the buttock, do not move your spine over it.

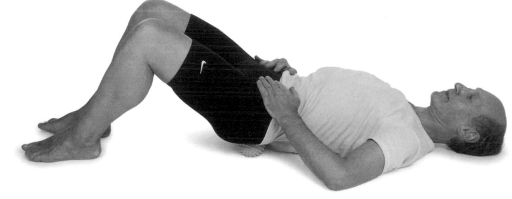

2 Repeat step 1, rolling the ball beneath your right buttock and moving over it to massage the muscles.

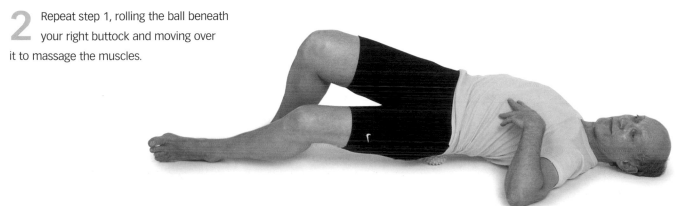

Level 1, Stage 1

An easy way of releasing tension, calming oneself, and achieving inner balance is to start each exercise session with a breathing exercise. If you hurry to get to a class on time, you may be anxious and a little breathless. After a few minutes of rhythmic breathing your heart rate and circulation slow, your skin cools and your emotions settle. Breathing is useful for regulating the physical effects of emotions. In these exercises, concentrate on letting the breath go and on building up a rhythm.

Achieving composure

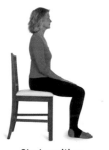

Start position
Sit comfortably on an upright chair, with your heels together and your feet against the floor.

You may need to work at the slow, controlled out-breaths in this exercise. They gradually increase in length, but they always require the same intensive effort. Practise this calming breathing exercise whenever you feel stressed. You can do it anywhere – in a traffic jam, in a crowd, on a commuter train.

1 Breathe gently in through the nose and out through the mouth, in through the nose and out through the mouth, to generate an even, spontaneous rhythm.

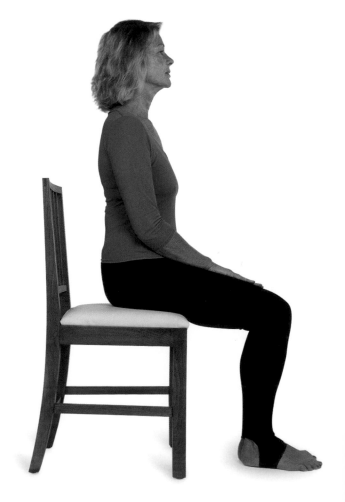

2 Slowly, breathing silently, count as shown below:

(...and 1... = a count of 1 second)

breathe in ... and 1 ... and 2 ... and 3 ...

breathe out ... and 1 ... and 2 ... and 3 ...

Repeat six times, or until your in-breaths and out-breaths are easy and controlled.

3 Keeping the in-breaths to three counts, gradually slow the out-breaths to four counts. Repeat six times.

breathe in ... and 1 ... and 2 ... and 3 ...

breathe out ... and 1 ... and 2 ... and 3 ... and 4...

4 Now, keeping the in-breaths to three counts, slow the out-breaths to six counts. Repeat four times.

breathe in ... and 1 ... and 2 ... and 3 ...

breathe out ... and 1 ... and 2 ... and 3 ...

and 4 ... and 5 ... and 6 ...

Countering immobility

This is an exercise to remember when you have to spend a long time sitting still. The strong down-push causes the leg muscles to contract, keeping the blood moving up to the heart and preventing it from pooling at the ankles. Breathe slowly and evenly, concentrating all your effort on the out-breath.

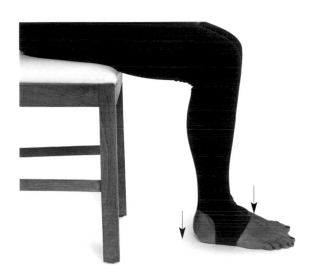

1 From the start position, breathe in while counting to three in an even rhythm. On the next out-breath, push both feet down hard and sustain the push for three counts. Repeat four times.

2 Breathe in for three counts. On the next out-breath, push both feet down hard and sustain the push for six counts. Sit taller on the slow out-breath.

3 Repeat step 2 until the pushes at the beginning of each repetition make a rhythm against the floor, and the movement is steady and strong on the slow out-breath.
It is easy to keep track of how many repetitions you have done if you count like this:

breathe in ...

one two, three ... out, two, three, four, five, six ...

two two, three ... out, two, three, four, five, six ...

three two, three ... out, two, three, four, five,

six ... and so on ...

Stability and mobility

Expressions relating to standing and using the feet, such as 'falling on one's feet' or 'having both feet on the ground' describe the quality of stability, which is the basis of movement. For example, when you push your feet down you activate the muscles of your legs and feet to move against the floor, producing a solid, strong stance. Pulling up from the waist to sit or stand tall shows how lightly one can sit or stand on two feet. Leg movements are minimized in these exercises, yet the leg muscles are exercised isotonically (the fibres do not shorten). The strong stance enhances awareness of the body, and this gives a sense of security that helps concentration.

The stabilizing down-push

You begin this exercise by pressing your feet down hard, and this brings you on to the sitting bones at the base of the pelvis. Be careful to apply equal force on both sides. For the push to work you have to press your heels together so you feel the inner muscles of your legs working, and your sitting bones against the seat. The muscles of the feet, the ankles, the legs up to the hips, and the buttocks all work together. Contracting the buttocks and thighs raises the body, so sit a little taller on each out-breath.

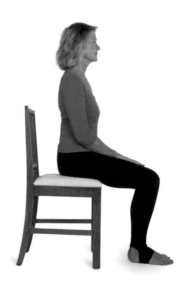

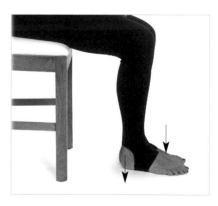

1 From the start position, breathe in while counting to three, press your heels together, push down with your feet, and breathe out to a count of three. Feel your leg muscles tighten and the sitting bones press against your seat. Repeat four times.

2 Breathe in for three counts, press your heels together, and push down for six counts. Breathe out slowly, feeling your feet against the floor and the sitting bones against the seat. Notice that your knees are apart. Relax completely. Repeat four times.

Shoulder roll

In this, the first of a series of exercises aimed at loosening the shoulder girdle, the action of placing the fingertips on top of the shoulders in step 1 opens the shoulders. It is an excellent way of testing the mobility of your shoulder girdle, for if it is stiff you will not be able to bring your elbows back while keeping your back straight. Practise two or three times a week, and you will soon find the tension easing and your shoulders moving back.

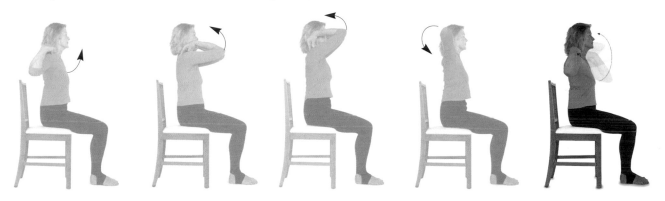

1 From the start position on page 88, breathe in, counting to three. On a slow out-breath, push down, contracting buttocks and thighs, to bring your trunk on to the sitting bones. Sit tall. Bending your elbows, raise your hands, palms open and turned up towards the ceiling, to shoulder level and put your fingertips on your shoulders in line with your ears.

2 Breathe in for three counts, and breathe out slowly for six counts while pushing your feet down. Feel your legs and lower stomach muscles help bring your pelvis to the correct angle of tilt (see page 31). Keeping your fingertips on your shoulders, bring your elbows forwards, towards the centre of your body.

3 Lift your elbows up parallel to your jaw, and slowly raise them (shoulders following) to your ears, then your temples, then to the crown of your head. Then on a slow out-breath, rotate them to point towards the back and around to the start position.

Rest and repeat

Relax, then repeat steps 1–3 slowly four times without a break, each time controlling the out-breath for a count of six. Then get up and walk around.

Repeat the shoulder roll four more times, then repeat it four times again, this time reversing the direction of the roll – you move your elbows up, back, lift them above your ears, and bring them forward and down. Then relax and walk around.

The sitting bones

When you sit, your weight rests on the bottom of the pelvic girdle, on two bony projections called the ischial tuberosities. For convenience they are called the 'sitting bones' in this book.

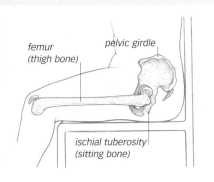

femur (thigh bone)

pelvic girdle

ischial tuberosity (sitting bone)

Getting the picture

Like the steps in a dance or the words in a play, exercises need
to be rehearsed, so that when practised the movements come
naturally. Rehearsing for an exercise involves going over it in your
mind so that each detail becomes imprinted on your memory.
This exercise shows you how to picture the step sequence as it
presents itself to you, and how to visualize its effects on your body.

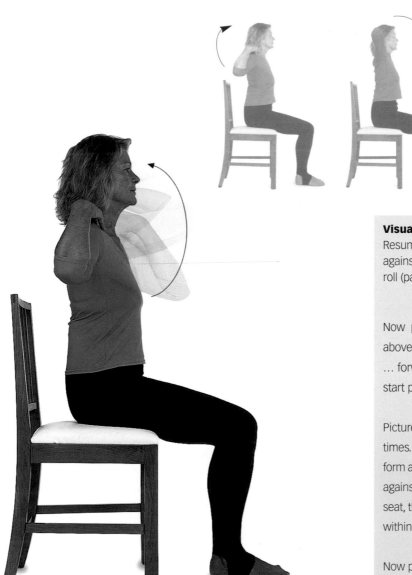

Visualisation

Resume the start position on page 88, feeling your sitting bones
against the chair seat. Close your eyes and review the shoulder
roll (page 91)… imagine yourself repeating each step.

Now picture yourself reversing the movements as illustrated
above … taking the elbows back … then up in line with the ears
… forward to meet opposite the nose … and down, back to the
start position.

Picture the shoulder roll four times more, then reverse it four
times. The effort of visualizing it with the eyes closed helps you
form an inner picture of the muscles involved, from the push down
against the floor, the buttocks and the sitting bones against the
seat, the back long, the neck balanced easily, the head poised – all
within a controlled out-breath.

Now practise the shoulder roll on page 91 twice while visualizing
the exercise, moving your arms in both directions.

Head, neck, and shoulders

A great deal of tension often resides in the shoulder area, and if it is allowed to persist the neck and shoulders become stiff, and posture may be affected. All the exercises on the next four pages help to loosen the trapezius muscle, the rhomboids, the lats and the pecs. How well you perform them will indicate how tight these structures have become, for these exercises take place against a wall, which becomes the measure of your success. If the mobility of your shoulder girdle is impeded by tension, you will be unable to pull both shoulders back against the wall while maintaining the correct alignment of the spine.

Using the wall

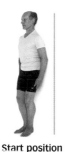

Start position
Start all the exercises on pages 94–97 standing with your back against the wall, your feet about 30 centimetres (12 inches) away from it, heels together, your knees slightly bent, and your hands by your sides.

The correct stance makes all the difference when you exercise against the wall. When you lean back against the wall in the start position, your shoulder blades and your seat touch it (1 and 2) but the back of your head does not (3), and neither does your middle back (4). Do check, however, that you are not arching your back. Bending the knees (5) straightens the back, as you can see from this photograph. Before beginning each exercise, check that you have not raised your chin (6) – your head needs to be upright, about 5 centimetres (2 inches) from the wall, and not tilting back. Your shoulders need to be relaxed and open, and your whole forearm (7), from elbows to hands, should rest against the wall.

Practise this stance before starting the next exercise, pushing both feet down, feeling your hands against the wall as you lift them, touching your shoulders with your fingertips, and visualizing them opening wide as you do so.

Points to watch

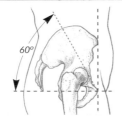

60°

■ Touching your seat against the wall helps tilt your pelvis at the correct angle (see page 31).

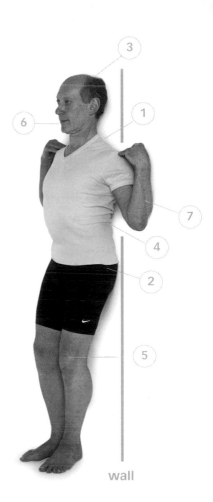

wall

Back-to-the-wall shoulder roll

This exercise will familiarize you with back-to-the-wall exercises. It is important to get the start position right, so begin by working slowly through the details illustrated on page 93. Keep your gaze level and your eyes focused ahead. Rather than check your position in a mirror, use your mind's eye. Stop when it feels right, and visualize yourself doing the exercise. Then follow the steps while visualizing yourself making each movement.

1 From the start position on page 93, take a short in-breath, press your heels together, and push both feet with even pressure against the floor. Open your shoulders and arms and lift your hands, touching your shoulders with your fingertips. Stretch up and look straight ahead.

2 On an out-breath, push down on your feet again, open your shoulders, and lengthen your back up against the wall. Feel the muscles contract at the sitting bones, and the lower stomach muscles lift to support the pelvis. Bring your

elbows forwards and slowly lift them above your ears, following with your shoulders.

3 Rotate your elbows outwards, and breathing out slowly, lower them, following with your shoulders and keeping them close to the wall, to the step 1 position.

Rest and repeat

Relax, close your eyes, and visualize the exercise. Walk around, then return and repeat steps 1–3 four times.

Points to watch

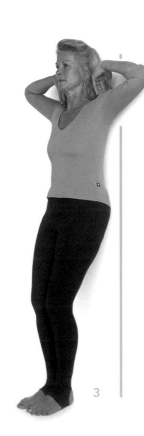

- In step 1, you press your lower back and tailbone against the wall and tilt your pelvis upright. But take care not to flatten your back and pull your navel flat against your spine, since this also tucks the tail under, which moves it away from the wall.
- Keep your shoulders down in steps 1 and 3, and keep your shoulders and chest open, as illustrated on page 93, throughout.

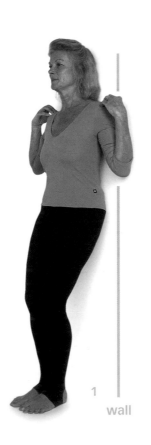

1

wall

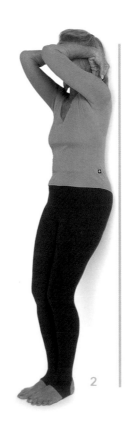

2

3

Back-to-the-wall owl head-swivel

Swivelling the head can be difficult until the upper body loosens and opens. It is important to keep the head upright, aligned with the wall but not touching it. Turn your head and neck gently – do not force them – leading with your eyes and keeping your gaze level and forwards, while turning through the upper back. As you touch your shoulders with your fingertips in step 1, open your chest.

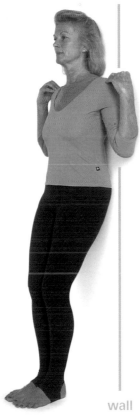

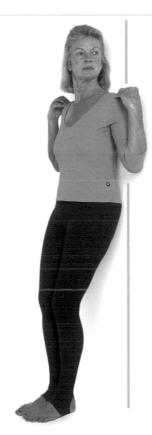

wall

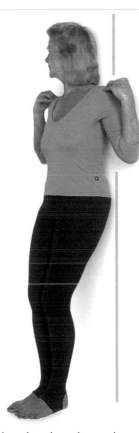

1 Adopt the start position on page 93, touch the tops of your shoulders with your fingertips, and pull down the lats so that your shoulders and elbows open towards the wall.

2 Push your feet down against the floor and feel your upright pelvis press your tailbone against the wall and your lower abdominal muscles lift to support your stomach. Lift your

upper back and neck, and on a slow out-breath turn your head toward your left shoulder, and back to the centre.

3 Breathe in and, breathing out slowly, turn your head to the right, and back to the centre.

4 Repeat steps 2 and 3 twice, and then relax.

Visualization

Picture yourself lengthening your back and neck and turning your head. Walk around and shake your shoulders. Visualize yourself moving naturally, without stiffness, then try to live up to this image of your movements.

Back-to-the-wall head and neck curl

Developing coordination in the upper body is the aim of this exercise, in which you curl down, stretching the spine vertebra by vertebra, until your eyes focus on your feet. It will counteract compression of the spine. Hold step 4 long enough to feel the stretch in your middle back and the extensor muscles of your neck and upper back stretch and lengthen.

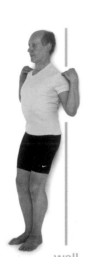 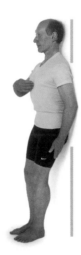 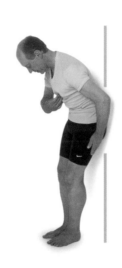 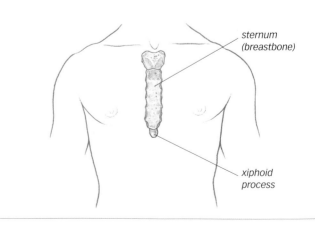

wall

1 Adopt the start position on page 93, touch your shoulders with your fingertips, open your shoulders, and push your feet against the floor. Feel your legs and the lower muscles of your stomach help tilt your pelvis to the correct angle.

2 Touch the xiphoid process with your right index finger, and think of it as the fulcrum of the movements your upper body makes.

3 With your chin down and your forehead leading, roll your head forwards and curl downwards, peeling your upper back away from the wall, towards your breastbone and a little beyond. Feel your middle back stretching.

4 Look at your toes and unroll slowly from your middle back to your fulcrum, to your upper back, to the back of your neck, then look straight ahead and open your shoulders.

Rest and repeat

Repeat steps 2–4 three times and then rest.

Xiphoid process

The small, leaf-shaped projection at the base of the sternum or breastbone is called the xiphoid process.

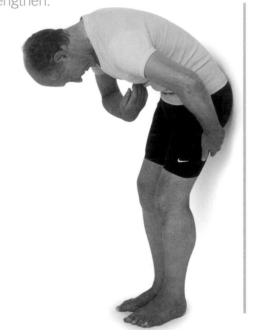

sternum
(breastbone)

xiphoid
process

Standing tall

Standing is an exercise in itself, for stance is never static. Through correct alignment and balance the skeletal structure is exercised against gravity. To achieve the ideal alignment think of the body as a number of elements stacked one on top of another. Consider the position of your pelvis and whether it is best placed to transmit the weight of your upper body to your feet. Are the curves of your spine aligned so as to minimize the weight of your head? Correct stacking of the body's skeletal elements is the basis of good posture, so instead of just standing upright, practise becoming practically and dynamically tall.

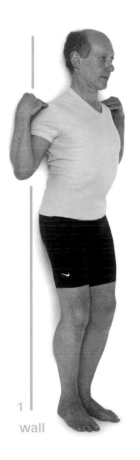

1
wall

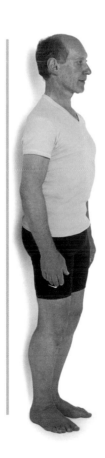

2

1 Stand in the start position on page 93, then widen your shoulders and place your fingertips on top of them, feeling your elbow, forearm and hand touch the wall. Slowly shift your feet back towards the wall until your heels are below your buttocks. Breathe in, and on a long, slow out-breath, press down equally on both feet. Close your eyes and picture your shoulders, open and relaxed, your fingertips resting on them, your head poised, your back and neck lengthened.

2 Without disturbing the picture in your mind's eye, lean forwards slightly, away from the wall. Push down on your feet and gradually straighten your knees so you stand tall and upright, your weight over your toes. Without changing your position, lower your hands to your sides and turn them so palms and fingers touch the sides of your thighs. Stand for a while, visualizing your stance.

3 Shake your arms and shoulders, then stand still, as natural and relaxed as possible. Think about the angle of your body: a little forward of the wall and not stiff and upright like a pole. Finish by walking around, keeping your stance natural and relaxed.

Opening the upper body

When the muscles of your chest stretch out, your back muscles contract; and when the back opens up, the chest is static. This natural balance is disturbed when one part of that action dominates. For example, people who do multiple sit-ups as part of their exercise routine often find that although their back opens up, the pectoral muscles of the chest tighten and they find it hard to move their shoulder blades. To restore the natural balance between the muscle groups of the upper thorax, these exercises stretch and then strengthen the muscles, front and back, restoring their natural range of movement by making them work. These are all wall exercises, but they are carried out facing the wall, and the wall becomes a part of the exercise.

Upper back stretch

This first exercise contracts the rhomboid muscles of the upper back and stretches the serratus anterior muscles, pulling the shoulder blades inwards. It is an intensive exercise, so go gently at first. When you are familiar with it and can perform it easily, however, you can make it more intensive by standing a little farther away from the wall and, in step 3, bringing the hands a little closer together but to the same height as before.

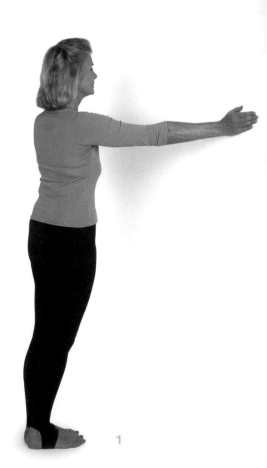

1 Stand facing the wall, about 45 centimetres (18 inches) away, with your heels pressed together. Stretch your arms out sideways, raising them to shoulder height and aligning elbows, palms and fingers with your shoulders.

2 Press your hands against the wall. Bend your knees and straighten your back, gently and as far as is comfortable, keeping your shoulders down and wide and your neck stretching up.

1

3 Breathe in while counting up to three, and push down equally with both feet against the floor. On the out-breath, bend your elbows and lean your trunk forwards as if it were hinged at the toes and ankles, allowing your heels to lift slightly. Bring your trunk closer to the wall, keeping shoulders and hips equidistant from it. Lift your elbows in line with your hands, keep your eyes focused straight ahead, and do not slide down against the wall. Move your shoulder blades closer together, then slowly push the wall away and stretch your arms out.

Rest and repeat

Pause and visualize the whole exercise, and repeat steps 1–3 four times, visualizing each step as you do it. Then relax and shake your body.

Shoulder blades

In step 3 the rhomboids contract, pulling the shoulder blades closer together and stretching the serratus anterior muscles, which form a thin muscle sheet from the sides of the ribs in front to the shoulder blades at the back.

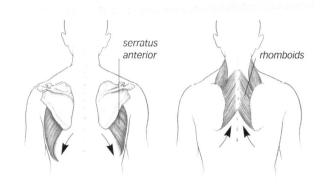

serratus anterior

rhomboids

Points to watch

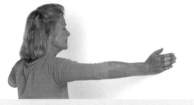

- Always remember to keep your elbows up, in line with your shoulders and hands.

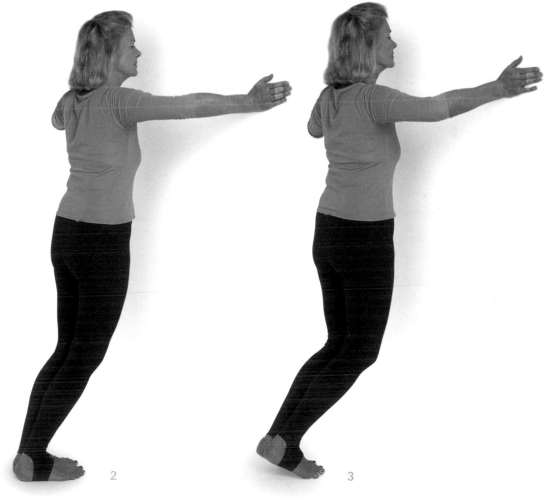

2

3

Up-the-wall shoulder and pectoral stretcher

Loosening tight pectoral muscles, which control the shoulder blades, and moving the arms forwards and down are the focus of this movement. It also stretches the front fibres of the deltoid muscles of the shoulders. Use the wall as a guide to progress. Keep your shoulders low and wide and your neck stretching up. After practising gently for a few weeks you should be able to get each shoulder in turn closer to the wall.

1

2

3

variation

1 Stand facing the wall, about 30 centimetres (12 inches) away, heels together, knees bent slightly. Lift your arms out to the sides and place your hands on the wall at shoulder height.

2 Breathe in counting to three, and on a slow out-breath, push down equally on both feet, pressing the heels together. Lean against your hands, and swivel your body left from your feet, looking to the left. Bend your left elbow and bring your right shoulder closer to the wall.

3 On a controlled out-breath, gradually take more weight on your left hand. Hold for a count of six, then rest.

Repeat and rest

Repeat steps 1–3, swivelling to the right. Then repeat the exercise on the left and the right three times, and rest.

Variation

To increase the level of difficulty, repeat steps 1–3 with your hand positioned higher up the wall, or lower down.

Points to watch

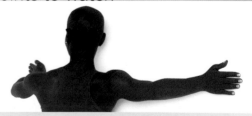

■ Increasing the weight on your left hand in step 3 brings your right shoulder closer to the wall, and stretches and straightens the inside arm and the right side of your chest and shoulder girdle.

Spinal spiral

Spiralling is one of the last movements to develop, and is the first we lose with time. One side tends to feel more stiff and tight than the other, and this maintenance exercise helps you check whether you are keeping stiffness at bay. You feel your balance spiralling from your knees up your spine to your neck as you work and loosen the middle back. It is an intensive exercise, so practise gently.

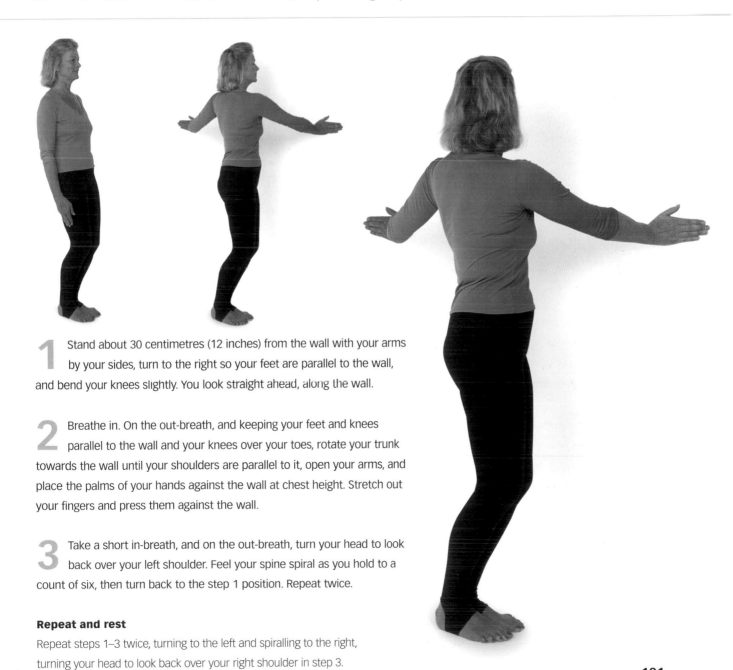

1 Stand about 30 centimetres (12 inches) from the wall with your arms by your sides, turn to the right so your feet are parallel to the wall, and bend your knees slightly. You look straight ahead, along the wall.

2 Breathe in. On the out-breath, and keeping your feet and knees parallel to the wall and your knees over your toes, rotate your trunk towards the wall until your shoulders are parallel to it, open your arms, and place the palms of your hands against the wall at chest height. Stretch out your fingers and press them against the wall.

3 Take a short in-breath, and on the out-breath, turn your head to look back over your left shoulder. Feel your spine spiral as you hold to a count of six, then turn back to the step 1 position. Repeat twice.

Repeat and rest

Repeat steps 1–3 twice, turning to the left and spiralling to the right, turning your head to look back over your right shoulder in step 3.

Waist stretcher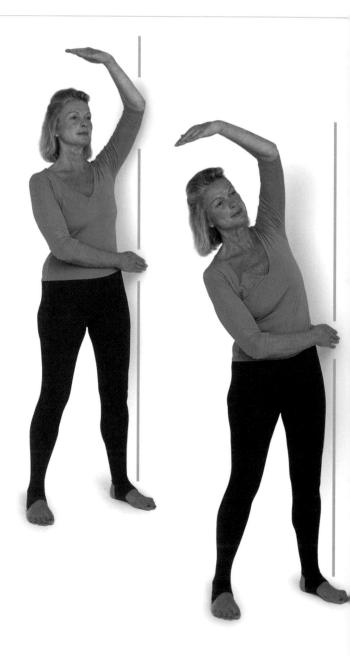

As well as the muscles of the waist, this exercise stretches the intercostal muscles that move the ribs. It corrects a common tendency to lift one hip higher than the other when walking, called 'hoisting the hip'. People who experience this find that one hip feels tighter than the other. Practise the following steps until the exercise feels easy, then repeat the stretch four times on each side. Keep the hip a uniform distance from the wall throughout the exercise – do not let it move away from or touch the wall.

1 Stand close to the wall facing right, your left foot touching the wall, your right foot 30 centimetres (12 inches) to the right of it, and your hands by your sides. Raise your left arm above your head and stand tall. Rest your right-hand fingertips against the wall, with your thumb touching your hip bone.

2 On an in-breath bend your knees slightly and press down equally on both feet. On the out-breath, reach up and away with your left hand, stretching your waist away from your hip bone. Keep your shoulders relaxed and open. Keep your head up, following the curve of your spine. Relax with your hands by your sides, then repeat the stretch twice.

Repeat and rest

Turn to face left, and repeat steps 1 and 2 three times.

Points to watch

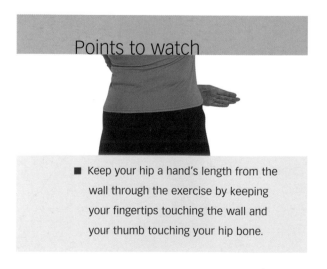

- Keep your hip a hand's length from the wall through the exercise by keeping your fingertips touching the wall and your thumb touching your hip bone.

Cat stretch

All the muscles that lower the shoulders are used in this exercise, which is performed up the wall. It stretches the upper back and thorax and lengthens the neck. Read through the exercise and visualize it step by step before doing it, then visualize it as you do it.

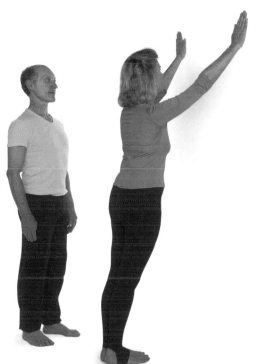

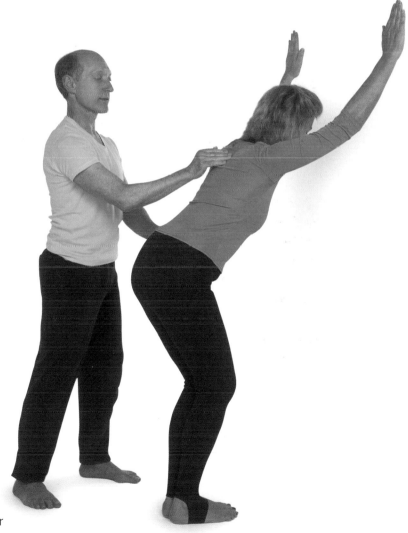

1 Stand facing the wall and about 60 centimetres (2 feet) away, with your heels pressed together. Raise both hands above your head, a little more than shoulder-width apart, and place them on the wall. Bend your knees to straighten your lower back.

2 Breathe in, counting to three, and on a slow out-breath, push down equally on both feet. Drop your shoulders, and pressing your hands lightly against the wall, lean close in to it, opening your chest, stretching your neck and your spine up, and pulling your hips and your tailbone away from the wall.

Repeat and rest

After you have worked through steps 1 and 2 once, repeat them four times. Then shake your shoulders to relax.

Up-the-wall push-ups

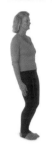

Start position
Stand facing the wall, ideally 60 centimetres (2 feet) from it – but if this seems hard, start 45 centimetres (18 inches) or even less away – with your shoulders wide, arms by your sides, palms touching thighs, and your knees slightly bent.

The following three exercises, called torso braces, are in fact push-ups made easy, but still effective for the upper body. They are strengthening exercises for the arms, which work in coordination with the whole torso. They also have the effect of evening out dominance of the left or right brain hemisphere. In time, they can be made more difficult by starting with the feet farther away from the wall. This loads more weight on the hands and increases the difficulty of supporting the torso and pushing it towards and away from the wall.

Push-up no. 1

This exercise works the shoulders, the pectoral muscles, and the lats. Instead of pushing your body away from the wall during step 2, think of yourself as pushing the wall away. This changes the emphasis, evening the body weight and making the action more controlled.

1 From the start position, turn your arms at the shoulders so the palms of your hands face forwards, fingers pointing to the floor. Keeping your shoulders open and your hands at thigh level, place your palms against the wall. Breathe in while counting to three, and push your feet down.

2 Bend your elbows and tuck them against you as you lean forwards from the balls of the feet, until your whole body from thighs to shoulders is parallel to the wall. On an out-breath and counting to six, brace yourself for the effort of pushing your hands against the wall to hold yourself against it, then push the wall away to lever yourself back to the step 1 position.

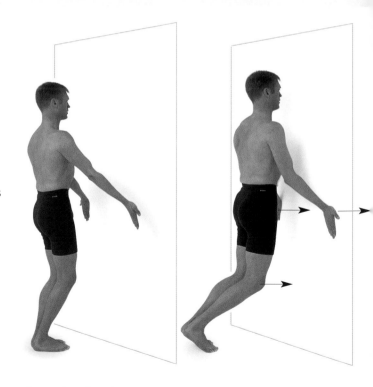

Repeat and rest
Repeat steps 1 and 2 as continuous push-ups four times, then rest.

Push-up no. 2

Strengthening the lats is the objective of this exercise, which can be the most difficult of them all. Concentrate on how you hold your torso while doing the push-ups, and on keeping the lats pulled down.

1 From the start position opposite, raise your hands and reach forwards, putting them against the wall at chest height, shoulder-width apart, fingers pointing up.

2 Breathing in on a count of three, push both feet with equal pressure down against the floor. On a controlled out-breath of six counts, lean your whole body forwards onto the heels of your hands, and, as your forearms move forwards to touch the wall, bring your elbows into your sides until they are in line with your hands. Pause, count to six, then lift away from the wall.

Repeat and rest

Repeat step 2 four times as a continuous sequence, then relax, shake your arms, and rest.

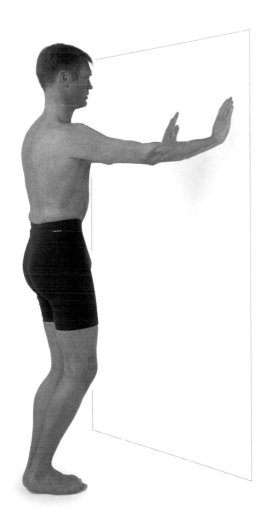
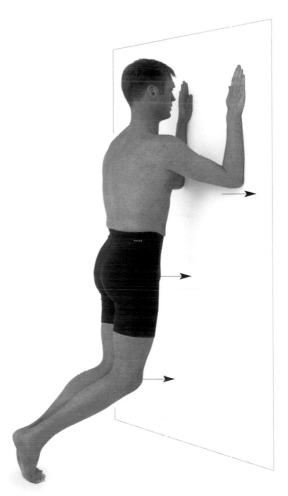

Push-up no. 3

Although this is an exercise for men and women, it is most popular with men who want to build up their pectorals and deltoids. It integrates the movements of the muscles of the shoulder girdle, and it stretches the whole torso. It makes you use your stomach muscles, because you move only your arms, keeping the rest of your body quite still. Breathe out as you lean in and push away, taking a short in-breath when you are upright.

1 From the start position on page 104, raise your hands, extend your arms above your head, and reach forwards to place your hands against the wall about 1 metre (3 feet) apart, lats and shoulders down, arms and fingers stretching up.

2 Take a short in-breath, and push both feet with equal pressure down against the floor. Now, on a slow, controlled out-breath, lean forwards, pause, and push the wall away so that your whole body from ankles to abdomen to head lifts as a unit away from the wall. Repeat and rest.

Points to watch

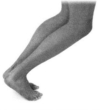

- Use your feet to stop yourself sinking down when pushing the wall away during step 2. Maintain your height by lifting your head and raising yourself on your ankles while pressing your feet down.
- Keep your pelvis still, pull up your abs, and do not arch your lower back.

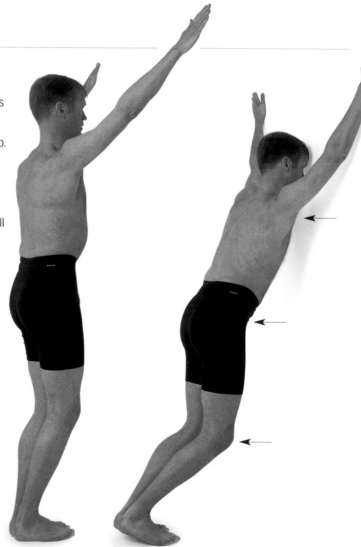

Repeat and rest

Repeat step 2 four times as an unbroken sequence of movements, then rest.

Arm movements

The arm is capable of a greater range of movement than the leg, yet turning the arm joint through its full range of movement is something people rarely do. These arm exercises integrate the movements of the muscles of the shoulder girdle, taking them through their full range sideways, above the head and back. Go gently at first: lack of use can stiffen the shoulder joint, and over-vigorous exercise is one cause of frozen shoulder, a condition in which the joint becomes painfully stiff.

Arm circle, palms up

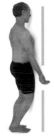

Start position
Stand facing the wall and close to it, with your toes touching the base of the wall and the palms of your hands against your thighs. Bend your knees so they touch the wall. Do not lean into the wall: your nose should be close but not touching it. Now pull your hips back so your trunk is parallel to the wall.

The shoulder joints have to swivel in their sockets to make this arm circle, because the palms of the hands are turned up. This mobility is easily lost, so this exercise might be difficult at first. Work at it to loosen the trapezius and levator scapulae muscles, which need to be pulled down, along with the lats. Keep your shoulders open. As your arms begin to circle, breathe out slowly, and take just a short in-breath before breathing out again.

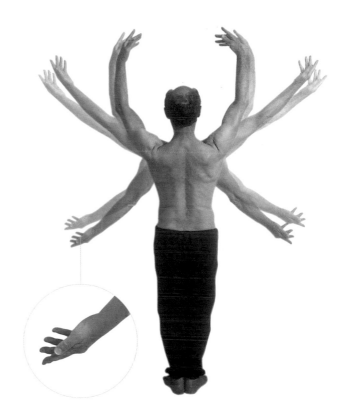

1 From the start position on page 104, open your arms from the shoulder joints so that your palms face the ceiling, and bend your elbows a little, holding your little fingers close to the wall. Breathe in, and then, breathing out as slowly as you can, draw a big half-circle with your fingers touching the wall from your thighs to high above your head.

2 Breathe in and on a slow out-breath reverse the movement in step 1, so you draw a half-circle from above your head back down to your thighs in one controlled movement.

Repeat and rest
Repeat steps 1 and 2 three times, then shake your body and shoulders and walk around.

Arm circle, palms away

In this second arm circle integrating exercise you turn the palms away from the body. Making a circle with the hands in this position is a little more difficult, so take it slowly and rest after each try. As the exercise gets easier, however, work through the steps several times in an unbroken sequence. These arm circles help you keep your shoulder joints mobile.

1 Adopt the start position on page 104, with the palms of your hands touching your thighs at the sides. Turn the palms outwards so your forearms and elbows face out, and open your shoulders.

2 On a slow out-breath, describe a half-circle with both hands, from your thighs to high above your head. Keep your shoulders open and stretch your neck up. Breathe in, and on the out-breath, slowly draw another half-circle with each arm from above your head back down to your thighs in one controlled movement.

Repeat and rest

Repeat steps 1 and 2 three times, then shake your body and shoulders, and walk around.

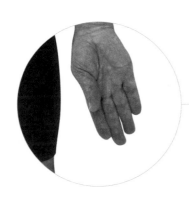

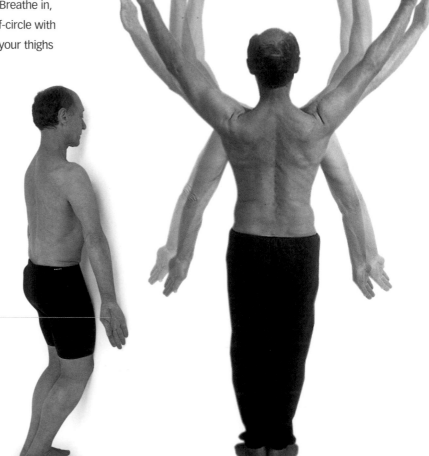

The flexible arm

The arm has more mobility than any other part of the body –
it can move through almost 360°. The shoulder bones
(the shoulder blade, the clavicle, and the humerus) can move
so freely because the cartilage capsule that surrounds the
joint (see page 33) is large and quite loose. The ligaments that
bind the bones together support and stabilize this joint, along
with the main shoulder muscles (the supraspinatus, the
infraspinatus, the subscapularis, and the teres minor) and
their tendons.

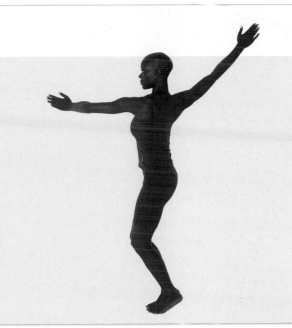

Triceps toner

This movement exercises the triceps muscles of the
arms. The backs of the arms at the top tend to go
flabby, especially in women, and this stretch is
especially effective for tightening this area.

1 Stand about 45 centimetres (18 inches) from the
wall and facing away from it, with your knees
slightly bent and your arms by your sides. Stretch your
arms back and keeping your hands roughly hip-width
apart, fingers pointing downwards, place your palms
against the wall behind you at about hip-height.

2 Lean your weight against the wall, open your
shoulders, and press on your hands, straightening
your arms. Stretch your whole body from the feet up.
Keep pressing and stretching to lift your body away from
the wall while breathing out slowly to a count of six.
Repeat six times, then rest your arms.

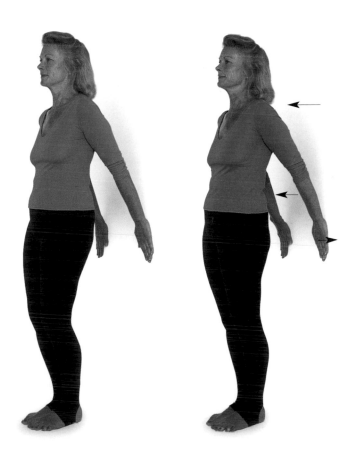

Legs and feet

The foot is remarkably flexible. The two arches formed by the long bones (see page 33) adjust to uneven surfaces during walking by twisting to the inside and the outside, so although the feet might become tired, the ligaments, muscles and tendons recover. In time, however, bad posture weakens these structures, which affects the lower back and, in turn, worsens the posture. The stirrup muscles (see page 57), which support the arch of the foot, are seriously affected by defects of posture. If overstretched, they cannot fulfil their function and the arches collapse. The foot exercises illustrated here strengthen the muscles of the feet and ankles, prevent the ankles from rolling inwards, and maintain the natural structure of the foot.

Foot rotations

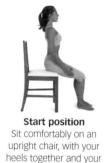

Start position
Sit comfortably on an upright chair, with your heels together and your feet against the floor.

Rotating the feet in different positions and directions strengthens the muscles of the feet and ankles, preventing collapsed ankles and arches. Pointing the feet strongly to work the arches sometimes causes foot cramps, however. To ease it, dorsiflex the foot or just walk around. Cramps sometimes occur when the muscles of the feet are not used to intensive exercise. After a few repetitions it recurs less frequently.

Pointing the foot

1 Lift the right leg, and breathe in. On the out-breath point the foot, and circle it from the ankle to the inside for four slow counts. Breathe in and on the out-breath circle it to the outside for four counts.

2 Push both feet against the floor and lift the left knee. Breathe out and repeat step 1, pointing the left foot and then circling it from the ankle to the inside, then to the outside, for four slow counts.

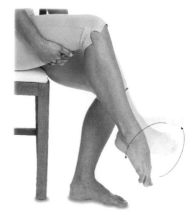

1

Flexing the foot

1 Push both feet down against the floor, then lift the left knee, placing your hands under the thigh to support the weight of the leg, and dorsiflex the foot – i.e. pull the toes up towards your knee. Try to keep the toes up while you circle the foot inwards from the ankle for four slow circles and reverse, circling outwards, for four slow circles.

2 Repeat step 1, this time lifting the right leg and rotating the right foot.

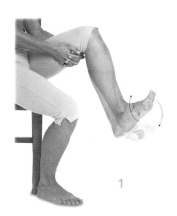

1

Strengthening the forefoot

The dorsiflexors of the foot – the muscles that bend it upwards – often become weak on the side where a knee or hip injury tends to throw the weight back on the heel. As a result, the forefoot is underused. This exercise rights the balance.

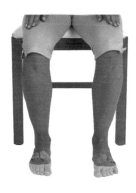

1

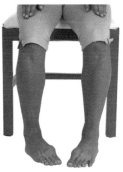

2

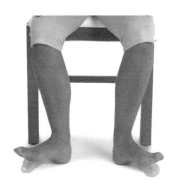

3

1 Sit in the start position and move the feet hip-width apart. Lift the arches of both feet, then press the toes and heels down.

2 Lift the feet from the ankle, turn them inwards, and tap the forefeet and toes on the floor,.

3 Lift the feet from the ankle, turn them outwards and tap the forefeet and toes on the floor.

4 Lift the feet, turn them to the front to resume the step 1 position and tap them on the floor.

5 Now repeat steps 2–4, tapping with both feet simultaneously and working up a good rhythm:

… feet pointing ahead … and up … and tap … and feet up and in … and tap … and up and out … and tap … and up and centre … and tap … and up and in … and tap … and up and out … and tap … and up and centre … and tap… and up …

6 When your shins tire, stop tapping, stretch the feet, and turn them to point ahead to rest them.

Simple leg dynamics

The muscles that bend the ankle, knee and hip joints need to be stretched to remain in condition, and the dynamic stretches on these two pages keep them flexible. They are load-bearing exercises to work the bones, and, because the rhythmic action of the leg muscles on the veins pumps blood and lymph upwards to the heart (see page 35), they speed circulation. Breathe in just enough air to be able to breathe out comfortably while counting slowly to six, and your next in-breath will be deeper.

Diving stance

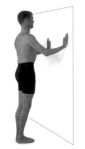

Start position
Stand about 30 centimetres (12 inches) from the wall, facing it, with the legs straight, the heels touching, and the feet nearly parallel. Stand tall (see page 97), and steady yourself with your hands against the wall.

This simple exercise engages all the major structures of the lower body, since as you push away from the ground, you use your body to counter gravity. It improves balance.

1 From the start position, spread your toes, and rest a fraction more of your weight on the forefoot and toes than on the heels. Lift those arches.

2 Breathing out to a count of six, bend your knees slightly and push down with equal pressure on both feet while pressing your heels together, as if about to dive off a springboard. Hold, keeping the knees slightly bent, and lifting from the hips while pushing down, then straighten your knees.

Repeat and rest
Repeat step 2 four times, controlling the movement on an even out-breath.

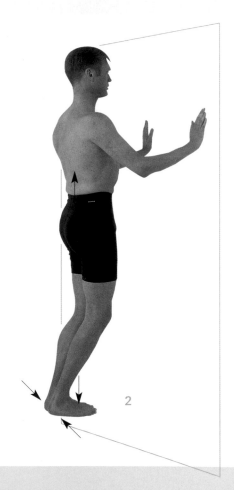

Visualization
As you begin step 2 of the Diving stance, and steps 1 and 3 of Knee bends and heel rises, opposite, picture your controlled out-breath opening and widening your shoulders. Imagine stretching your spine upwards against a wall, lengthening it and freeing your neck.

Knee bends and heel rises

This exercise strengthens the complex muscle structure of the knee joint and works the quadriceps and hamstrings in the thigh, which tighten if underused. It reduces hyperextended knees, exercises the muscles of the calves and ankles, and improves balance. Begin slowly, and gradually work up to repeating the bends and stretches for several minutes.

1 From the start position on page 112, bend your knees, checking that they are in line with your toes, and move your weight forwards onto the forefeet without lifting your heels. Take an in-breath, and breathing out slowly to a count of six, push down equally on both feet, pressing your heels together and down against the floor.

2 Take a short in-breath, and breathing out slowly to a count of six, straighten your knees, feeling the stretch all the way up your legs.

3 Breathe in, rise on to your toes, and on a slow, controlled out-breath stretch from top to toe.

4 Breathe in and on a slow out-breath, lower your heels to the floor. Stay tall as you press both feet down, and feel the stretch from hip to ankle. Hold, then relax and shake your legs.

Repeat and rest
Repeat steps 1–4 slowly, then repeat them ten times, making a rhythm of pushing down, bending and straightening the knees, and raising and lowering the heels. Then relax and walk around.

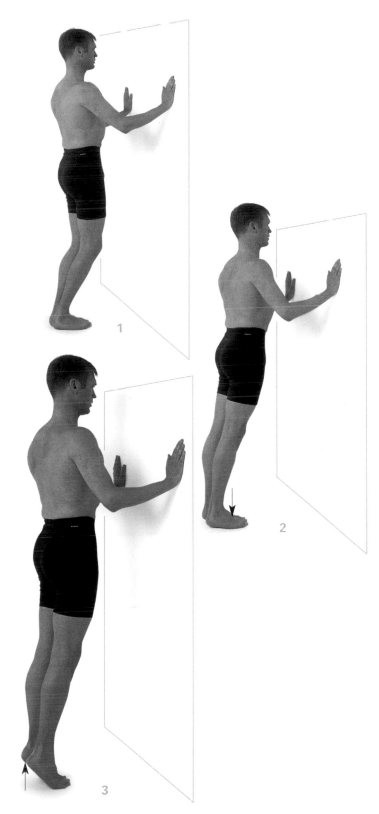

Calf stretches

This exercise will ease tightened calf muscles, which may result from lack of exercise or from wearing high-heeled shoes. They restore the natural position of the foot and improve balance. Do not force the stretch, however, and do not bounce when stretching, because this can tear the muscles.

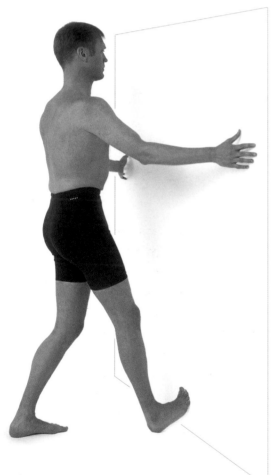
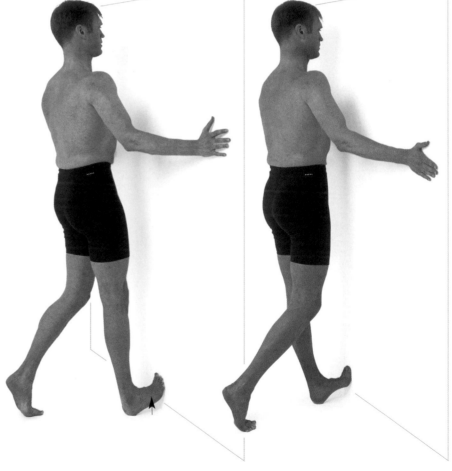

1 Stand 45 centimetres (18 inches) from the wall in the start position on page 112. Bend your knees, lift your right foot, and move it forward to press the lifted toes against the wall. The bent front knee should be over the toes, and the back foot aligned with the back hip.

2 On a long out-breath, gently stretch the calf by straightening the front leg. As you feel the stretch, move both hips forward by pushing on the ball of the back foot until the heel rises. Keep the heel of your front foot still and do not let your toes slide down.

3 Repeat steps 1 and 2 twice, then step forward with the left foot and repeat the exercise three times.

Hips and thighs

Everyone worries at times about muscle tone in the hips and thighs. However, some hip muscles have a structural role in maintaining the balance of the body, so they must be worked on first. They may be shortened due to underuse, and need to be stretched before they can be toned. Trying to improve the tone of shortened muscles runs the risk of overstretching and causing minor injury, which can have a detrimental effect on the balance of the whole body. These exercises stretch the hip flexors and the hamstrings at the backs of the thighs, and they loosen the pelvic area in preparation for the Level 2 exercises, which work on toning the thighs and the buttocks.

Forward bend

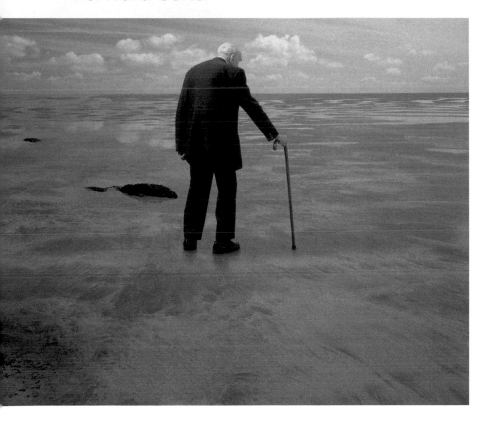

People usually think a weak spine is to blame for a bent-over posture in later life. People – women especially – who suffer from osteoporosis often develop a dowager's hump because of bone loss in the spine. However, the bent-over posture characteristic of old people is often the result of lifelong poor posture: many people in their twenties have a pronounced stoop. In time, this bad habit weakens the hip flexors and the muscles that support the lower back, stretches and weakens the muscles of the upper spine, and keeps the muscles that move the shoulders rigid, making it difficult to pull the shoulders back.

If you spend much of your time sitting and never stretch the hip flexors, they may tighten permanently. In time, this can cause a bent-forward posture.

Hip flexor stretch

This exercise stretches the hip flexors – the muscles that bend and straighten the legs from the pelvis. If you have to sit for prolonged periods at work these muscles get very tight, causing you to bend forwards. If you have painful toe joints place the foot of the leg you stretch back on a cushion positioned behind you for support.

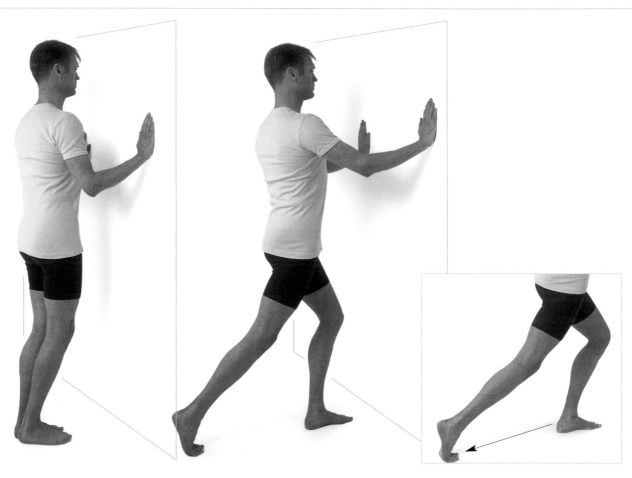

1 Stand about 30 centimetres (12 inches) away from and facing the wall, and steady your body with your hands. Stand upright with your knees aligned over your toes, and move your weight forwards, over your knees.

2 Bend your knees and free your right foot to take one step back. On an out-breath, gently deepen the bend in the front knee to stretch the right hip and thigh. Stretch up from the hips, feeling the stretch along the thigh of the back leg. Push down with the back foot to increase the stretch.

3 Take the back foot farther back, resting the weight on the ball of the foot, while bending the front knee a little more. Hold, then resume the step 1 position and change legs.

Repeat and rest
Repeat steps 1–3, this time taking the left leg back, then rest.

Alternative hip flexor and hamstring stretch

The hamstrings at the back of the thighs are often never stretched. This multipurpose exercise is an alternative hip stretch to the one opposite. It stretches the fronts and the backs of the thighs and lifts the buttocks, and it is good for stiff knees. From step 1, check that your legs are aligned: the knees in line with the hips and the ankles.

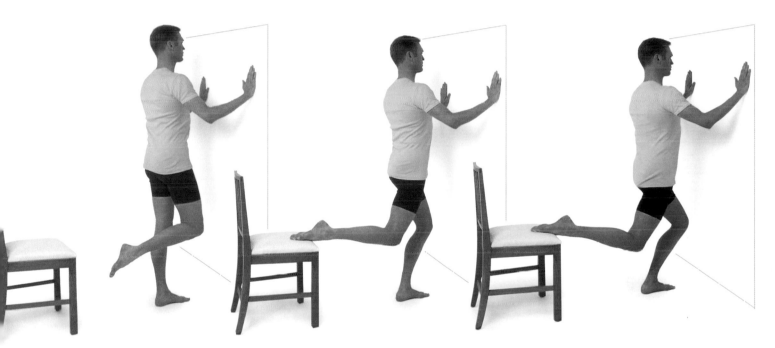

Points to watch

■ For better control and greater comfort when supporting one leg on the chair seat, rest your shin and the instep of your foot on the seat.

1 Stand facing and about 30 centimetres (12 inches) from the wall, with an upright chair placed a comfortable distance behind, the seat facing the wall. Steady yourself with both hands against the wall, then bend both knees and raise your right foot.

2 Put the instep of the right foot over the edge of the chair seat, and on a slow out-breath, gently bend the supporting knee to stretch the right thigh and hip flexors.

3 Repeat the stretch for three long out-breaths, deepening the stretch on the supporting leg, then stand up straight as at the beginning of step 1.

Repeat and rest

Repeat steps 1–3, this time stepping back with the left foot and bending the left knee.

Thigh and hip-flexor stretch

As well as stretching the hip flexors and the psoas, this exercise stretches the ankles and makes the knees more flexible. The movements are gentle: you simply bend each knee in turn by placing the foot on a chair seat; but go carefully if your knees are stiff.

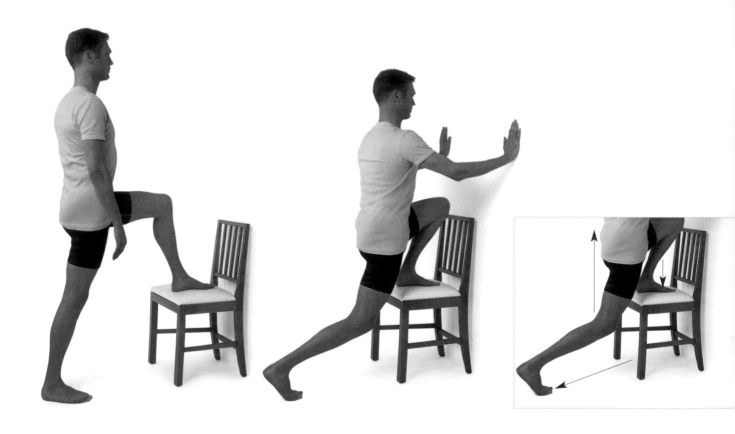

1 Stand facing an upright chair. Free your left leg, lift the foot, and place it on the chair seat.

2 Lean forwards to place your hands against the wall for support. Push your feet down, one against the floor, the other against the chair seat. Breathe out as you stretch the front of your right thigh. Keep your hips in line and think of lifting your upper body out of your waist.

3 Now move the right foot farther back to get a deeper stretch over the hip above it and in the hamstrings of the bent leg. Breathe out to a count of six, pushing both feet down. Repeat this step twice.

Repeat and rest

Repeat steps 1–3, this time placing your right foot on the chair seat.

Thigh and knee stretch

Some people find it difficult to bend a knee up behind the back, and this stretch will help you to get there. If, when you try it, your knee feels uncomfortable, return to the knee bends on page 113, and try this exercise again when your quads feel more stretched.

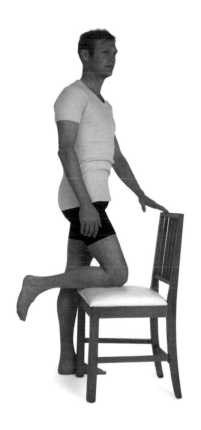
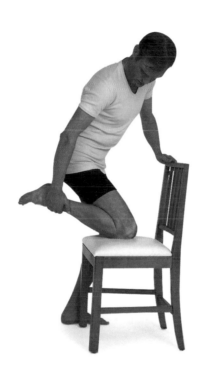
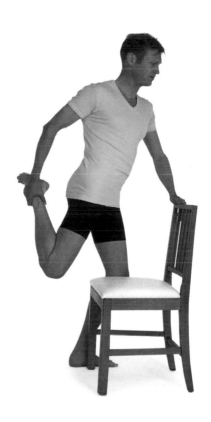

1 Stand facing the seat of a high-backed chair, then move it to your right side. Holding the back with your left hand for support, bend your right knee and place the shin on the chair seat. Now make a half-turn to your right and stand comfortably with all your weight on your left leg.

2 Bend your left leg and relax downwards. Raise your right heel and at the same time grasp your right ankle with your right hand to support it from beneath, pulling it upwards to touch your right buttock. Slowly raise your hips until your left leg supports all your weight.

3 On a slow out-breath, and keeping your right thigh and knee in line with your right hip, push down with your right foot against your right hand to increase the stretch still farther. Repeat three times.

Repeat and rest

Repeat steps 2 and 3, this time moving the chair to your left, and holding your left foot with your left hand to stretch the thigh and knee.

Lower back and thigh stretch

This chair squat gives the lower trunk and upper legs a good stretch. Press your heels hard together. Holding on to a chair provides a counterbalance and gives you a degree of control as you let yourself down. If your knees feel stiff, go easy and do not squat too low.

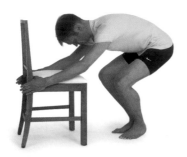 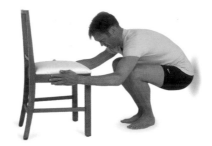 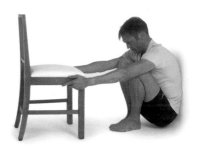

1 Stand facing a chair, with your back about 30 centimetres (12 inches) from a wall, heels together. Bend your knees, bend forwards, and stretch out to grasp the chair back.

2 Breathe in and on a slow out-breath, squat down as far as you comfortably can, supporting your lower back against the wall. Hold, counting to six, then rise slowly to stand up.

3 Repeat step 2 four times, squatting more deeply each time. On the last repetition your hands should grasp the front of the chair and your seat almost touch the floor. Then rest.

Bear stance

Give your lower back the best preparation for stretching by bending your trunk as low as you can before kneeling in the bear stance. Your left knee does not quite touch the floor in step 3.

1 Sit on a chair with your legs and feet parallel, your heels touching and your hands on your knees.

2 Lean forwards and place your hands shoulder-width apart on the floor. Breathe in.

3 On a long out-breath, move your hands forwards and lower your knees close to the floor. Hold for a count of six, then walk your hands back towards your knees, raise your knees and hands, and sit back on the chair.

Repeat and rest

Rest briefly, then repeat steps 1–3 four times, and relax.

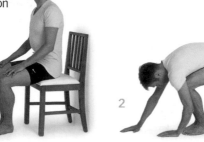 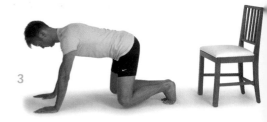

1

2

3

Bear stretch

When you can perform the bear stance easily, you are ready to
move on to the bear stretch. This exercise really tests whether you
can stretch the backs of your legs. If you find it impossible at first,
persevere. Regular practice produces amazing results, so that within
a month you will find the muscles of your calves, hamstrings and
back stretching farther than you ever thought they would. After
each try, walk around and shake the body well. When you feel you
have mastered it, continue to practise it two or three times a week
to keep your hamstrings stretched.

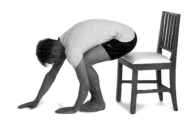 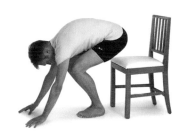 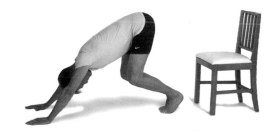

1 Sit in the step 1 position for the Bear stance on
page 120, breathe in, stretch forwards, and place
your hands shoulder-width apart on the floor.

2 On a slow out-breath, push your hands and feet
down on the floor, bending your knees.

3 Raise your heels and hold the position as long
as is comfortable, then walk your hands back
towards your knees and sit back on the chair.

Repeat and rest
Repeat steps 1–3, then relax and rest.

Variation
Repeat the exercise often, stretching in the step 3 position for
longer and longer until you can hold it for 3 minutes, pushing
down on your hands and feet as you breathe out. Push your
heels down and walk your hands closer to your feet,
straightening your knees. Eventually you will be able to place
hands and feet together flat on the floor.

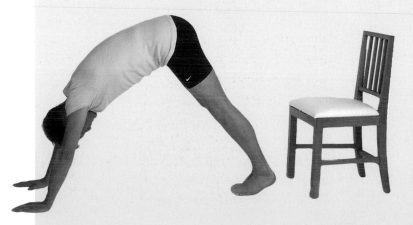

Stretching out and pulling in

Like rugby football players out on the field, you stretch the abductor muscles in your hips (which move your legs outwards) and exercise the adductor muscles (which pull them back in) in the next three short exercises. Go as low as you can in the first exercise, below, and make your legs active by opening them wider in the second. The third exercise, on page 124, works both sets of muscles and can help correct a misaligned kneecap.

Working the hip muscles

Begin this exercise with your feet about 1 metre (3 feet) apart. When it begins to feel easy you can increase the difficulty by gradually moving your feet wider apart.

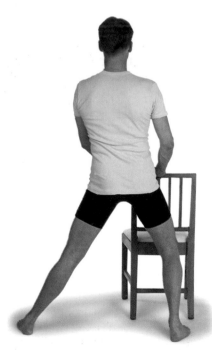 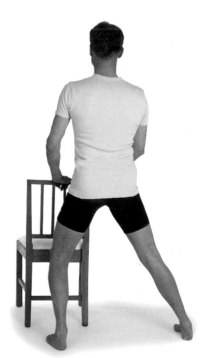

1 Stand behind a chair with your feet apart, toes pointing forwards, and your hands on the chair back. Move your left foot farther to the side to widen the stance, then lunge to the right. Hold at the lowest point that still feels comfortable. Return to the centre.

2 Repeat step 1, this time moving your right foot farther to the side and lunging to the left.

Repeat and rest

Repeat the exercise several times, then rest.

Knee strengthener

If you feel pain underneath your kneecap when walking, it may be because the kneecap does not track in a straight line from the knee bent to the knee straight position, and that the femur and tibia bones that meet at the knee joint are misaligned. The quadriceps muscles of the thigh bend and straighten the knee, but if the vastus medialis muscle on the inside of the thigh (see page 161) is underdeveloped, the kneecap veers to the outside and scrapes over the heads of the femur and the tibia. Exercising the affected knee as shown here works this muscle. Repeat the exercise frequently to build it up quickly.

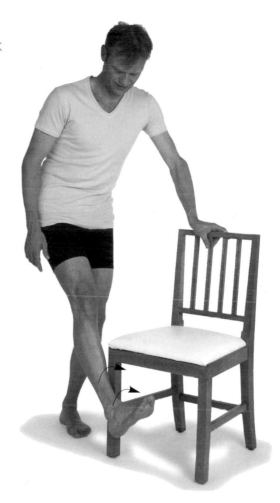

1 Stand behind a chair and press your hands down on the chair back. Flex the foot of the affected leg upwards and turn it inwards.

2 Straighten the knee and press the side of your foot inwards against the chair leg. Feel the muscles above the knee contract, especially the weak inside one. Hold for a count of six, then rest and repeat.

Kneecap tracking

When the leg is straightened, the kneecap moves over the knee joint and slides up, down and even sideways between the tendon of the quads and the patellar ligament, which binds the tendon to the knee joint. When the quads tighten, the kneecap helps lock the knee. When the quads pull evenly, the kneecap tracks straight up and down, as shown by the arrows.

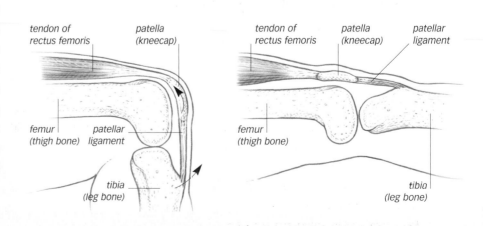

Activating the legs

The first stage of Level 1 exercises ends with this floor exercise
to work the adductors in step 2 and, in step 3, the abductors.
Rest your head on a cushion to keep it aligned with your spine.

1 Lie on your back, bend your
knees, and place your feet side
by side on a cushion. Press your lower
back down to keep your pelvis flat.

2 Open your thighs sideways from
the hip joints and press the soles
of your feet together. On an out-breath,
tense the adductor muscles that move
your thighs inwards, imagining you are
holding a weight on the inside of each
knee. Hold for a count of six, and relax.
Repeat six times, then return to the
step 1 position and rest.

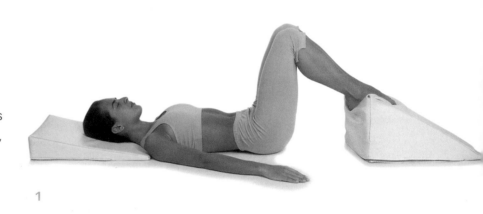

1

3 Open your thighs as wide as you
can, then keeping your lower
back flat on the mat, work your
abductor muscles to push your knees
still further down. Repeat six times.
Resume the step 1 position, and rest.

Repeat and rest
Repeat steps 1–3 six times, then roll on to
your side to get up, and walk around.

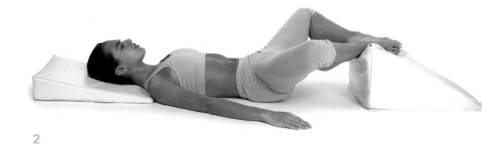

2

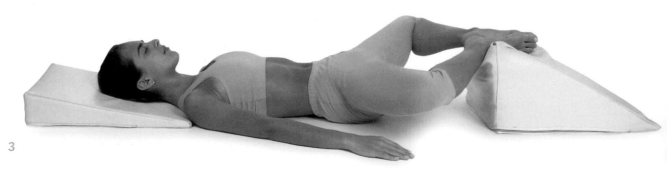

3

124

Level 1, Stage 2

In ports and industrial cities everywhere, passersby sometimes see trucks and automobiles hoisted by crane. Each one has a different loading, and to achieve the delicate balance needed for lifting, its centre of gravity has to be found. For the purpose of exercising the human body, it is necessary to think of it in similar terms: as a unit with a centre of balance. The best way to suspend it in the air would be to invert it into the position for a backbend, because a cable attached to a specific pivotal point between the hips would turn the inverted body into a perfectly balanced unit for hoisting. This pivotal midpoint in the pelvis is the body's natural centre of gravity and its working centre. Keeping its structures toned and flexible is of longstanding benefit.

The body's pivotal point is the spot where a straight line from the top of the head to the feet crosses a horizontal line drawn between the hips when standing (see page 135). The lines cross in the lower part of the pelvis, called the pelvic floor. When they are strong and healthy, the central stabilizing muscles of the pelvic floor anchor and balance the body. However, because this is not an area of skeletal muscle with tendons that act on joints to move muscles, we are scarcely aware of it. Only dancers, acrobats and the like, dependent for technique on the integration of skeletal balance and pull, normally worry about the location of their pivotal centre.

Yet, at some point every body will demand special attention to the waist and the lower back. In neglected bodies of all ages, signs of the pelvic floor's off-centre shift, such as the pot belly and lower back pain, are always noticed and usually lamented. The sit-up, usually thought of as the cure-all exercise for postural defects, often makes things worse, since it creates an imbalance between muscles supporting the abdomen and those supporting the spine internally.

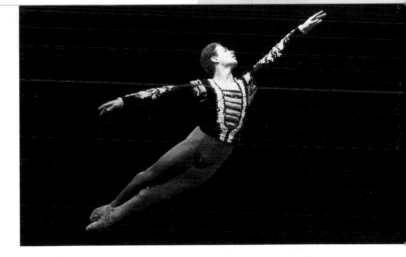

Finding the midpoint – the body's practical working centre – and exercising to maintain its strength and keep it in its natural position, helps dancers execute gravity-defying leaps with grace and accuracy.

These effects are not unavoidable, however. They are not inevitable signs of ageing as is commonly supposed. What is needed is perseverance in learning how to rehabilitate and strengthen the pelvic floor and restore its contribution to the body's natural balance. The exercises in Level 1, Stage 2 concentrate on exploring this important area of the body.

Wake-up

A breathing exercise before beginning each practice session eases the transition between everyday preoccupations and the concentration needed to carry out the exercises effectively. The breathing exercise that introduces Stage 2 is heady and strenuous if carried out correctly, but it energizes the body and relaxes and composes the mind. The 'wake-up' exercises shown on the next three pages prepare the body for the important pelvic floor exercises that follow by stretching and exercising the often under-used muscles of the lower abdomen. Before beginning each exercise, read through the steps and imagine doing the movements.

Exercising the heart and lungs

This exercise works the heart and lungs hard, so be sure to rest and recover before repeating it. Do it only once or twice a day to start with, but gradually increase the repetitions to ten.

1 Sit on an upright chair with your feet almost parallel, heels touching, and knees open opposite your hips. Your arms hang either side of the chair, palms facing forwards. Take a short in-breath, and on the out-breath, push both feet down against the floor, and bring your hands, palms facing the ceiling, up from your sides in a wide circle to reach above your head.

2 Hold your hands high for a few seconds, still pushing down on the chair seat and on the floor, then breathe in and press the palms of your hands together above your head, holding your breath for a count of six.

3 While holding your breath and keeping your palms pressed together, slowly bring your hands down to your lap, fingers pointing to the floor, then breathe out strongly.

Repeat and rest

Give yourself time to recover, then repeat steps 1–3. After you finish, walk around for a minute and shake your arms and legs.

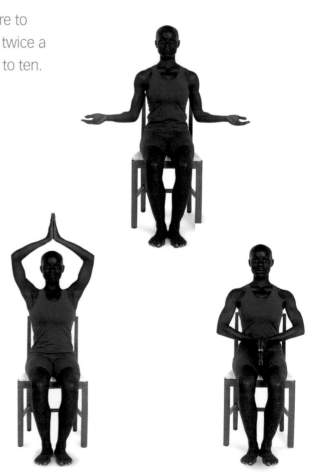

Sitting tall

This posture, along the lines of Standing tall on page 97, is designed to wake up and start toning the muscles of the lower abdomen, especially the transversus abdominis. It also works the triceps muscles, which straighten the upper arms. Concentrate on keeping the lower back straight – lean back at an angle about 80° from the floor, but keep it in line with the upper spine. Keep your head upright throughout, your eyes facing forwards.

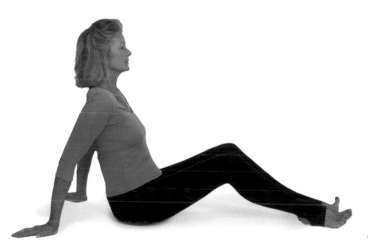 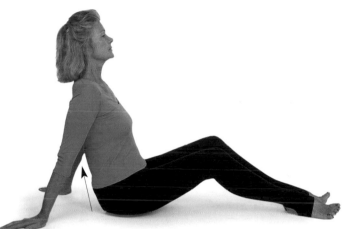

1 Sit on the floor with your knees slightly bent and parallel, in line with your hips, and your hands on the floor behind your sitting bones. Press the sides of your feet together, and push your heels into the floor so that the forefoot rises from the floor.

2 Pull up your buttock muscles so you sit upright on the sitting bones. Take a short in-breath, and on a long, slow out-breath, press both hands down on the floor, straighten your elbows, and lean back at an angle of about 80° from the floor. Pull your lats down, and open your shoulders. Sit up from your sitting bones to stretch your spine and neck. As you continue to breathe out, you feel the muscles of your lower abdomen pull towards your lower back to support the body at that angle.

Points to watch

- Tighten your lower abdominals as you lean back in step 2. Do not arch the lower back.
- Keep your seat balancing on the sitting bones throughout. Do not let it slide forwards.
- Keep your shoulders down and back.

Rest and repeat

Relax and sit forwards on the next in-breath, and repeat step 2 four times.

Introducing the obliques

This variation on Sitting tall on page 127 has the same purpose: to awaken the abs, but it includes an abdominal contraction and also stimulates the external and internal oblique muscles of the abdomen. Begin in the same position as for Sitting tall.

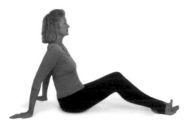

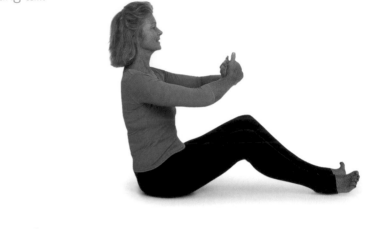

1 Repeat steps 1 and 2 of Sitting tall on page 127, and keeping your palms pressing down against the floor, lean back from the sitting bones at a slight angle.

2 Still leaning back, bring the palms of your hands together below your chest. Take a short in-breath, and on the out-breath, press your palms together, tighten your buttock muscles to lift up on your sitting bones, and draw your lower stomach muscles towards your back.

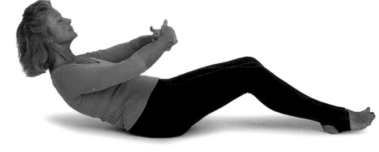

3 Curl back from the sitting bones and the low back to intensify the contraction in the centre of the lower abdomen. Stop when this feels strong and effective, and remain in this position for three slow out-breaths.

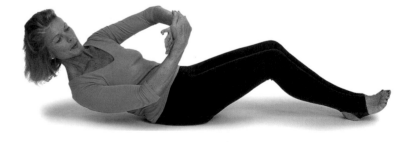

4 Rotate your trunk towards the right from the waist to engage the obliques. Hold for three slow out-breaths.

5 Now rotate to the left to work the obliques on the other side for three slow out-breaths.

Repeat and rest

Now repeat the exercise, keeping your neck stretching up as you lean back. Rest, then get up and walk around.

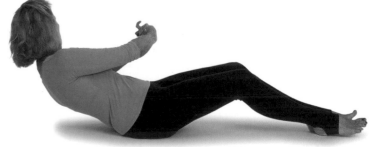

The pelvic floor

I am always surprised to see how little emphasis exercise teachers, sports trainers, and even athletes and dancers place on the pelvic floor. Most mothers have learned a few pelvic floor exercises during antenatal classes, but when they begin pilates many of my clients are only dimly aware that they have a pelvic floor. Some of the men have to be persuaded that their pelvic floor is a movable part of the body, and are astonished when I explain that it needs exercise, just like the biceps and other muscles. Even trained dancers may not fully understand the role of the pelvic floor muscles in carriage and movement, yet to anyone with a trained eye, their influence is clear in the way dancers stand, balance and elevate.

Your pelvic floor is such an important structure that to let it lose tone and elasticity is to throw your whole body out of alignment. Your pelvic tilt is lost, your posture sags tellingly, your abdomen protrudes, and the muscles that control your rectum and bladder, and your vagina if you are a woman, weaken.

The pelvic floor is a thin membrane or diaphragm made up of layers of muscle and connective tissue suspended across the pelvic girdle. Above it are the organs of the abdomen: the intestines, the rectum and bladder, and, in women, the womb. Without the diaphragm, they would fall or 'prolapse' through the opening in the centre of the pelvic girdle. The pelvic floor is funnel-shaped, so the pressures on it are all downward-directed, but it is a dynamic structure, normally strong and elastic enough to support the abdomen. Its outer muscles surround the external sex organ in men and the vagina and clitoris in women, and so help sustain libido. The exercises on these next few pages help you use your pelvic floor muscles and make you more conscious of your centre of balance.

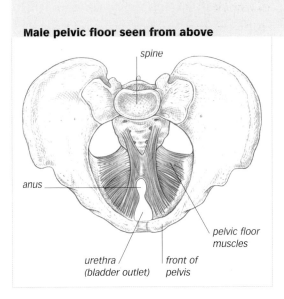

Male pelvic floor seen from above

spine

anus

pelvic floor muscles

urethra (bladder outlet)

front of pelvis

The pelvic floor is as important to men as to women. This diagram looks down on the muscles of the male pelvic floor. Involving your pelvic floor muscles as you exercise protects the lower back and stops you straining your abdominal muscles when you lift heavy objects. It makes you move more efficiently and exercise more effectively.

Making the connection

If you are not used to exercising your pelvic floor it can be hard at first to find the muscles to move. If they have lost tone they do not seem to respond to attempts to move them. Because most of the pelvic floor is inside the body, your eye cannot see it move and only your mind's eye will tell you whether you are making the right movements. A good way to start is through breathing exercises, because the internal muscles of the pelvis are closely linked to the respiratory diaphragm, the muscle that controls the flow of air into and out of the lungs. In the exercise opposite, visualization, combined with a strong down-push with the feet (see page 89) will help you to get a feeling for the muscles involved, and to move them rhythmically.

The breathing connection

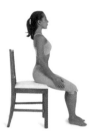

Start position
Sit near the front edge of an upright chair with your heels touching and your feet almost parallel. Open your shoulders and rest your hands lightly on your thighs. Relax and breathe normally.

In this exercise you concentrate on breathing, focusing on the out-breaths. It omits the down-push on the feet, which you practised in most of the Stage 1 exercises.

1 On a long, even out-breath, lengthen your trunk from the sitting bones, and the spine from the tailbone, without collapsing the chest, and raise your head.

2 Take a short in-breath, close your eyes, and breathe out for as long as you can. Notice your shoulders widen, your spine and neck lengthen, your rib cage narrow from armpits to waist, and your lower stomach muscles gradually pull across to support the contents of the abdomen.

Repeat and rest
Take in enough air for the next out-breath, and repeat step 2. Then rest and repeat the exercise four times.

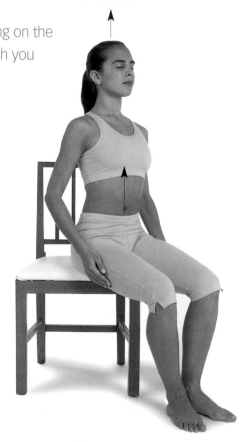

The body/mind connection

In this exercise, pushing down with the feet, lifting on to the sitting bones, and contracting the buttocks against the chair makes you lift up inside; and the sensation of lengthening from tailbone to head gives an image behind closed eyes of lifting off. Start each step by visualizing it, then put it into practice.

1 From the start position opposite, balance on the sitting bones against the chair seat and push both feet with equal pressure against the floor. Take a short in-breath, relaxing your stomach muscles and pelvic floor muscles gently downwards.

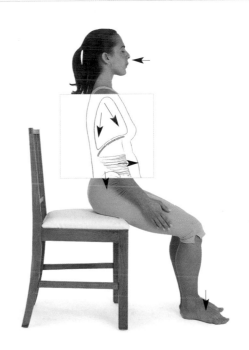

2 Breathe out slowly, visualizing the muscles between your tailbone and pubic bone rising, then lifting them. As your breath runs out, use your abdominal muscles to draw down the respiratory diaphragm, emptying the lungs further. Continue to lift your pelvic floor, and feel the tranversus abdominis muscles of your lower stomach pull across and inwards.

Rhythmic breathing

Breathe out again slowly, visualizing the muscles between tailbone and pubic bone rising, then lifting them. On the in-breath, relax your stomach muscles and pelvic floor gently downwards again. Then repeat steps 1 and 2 four times, breathing out slowly and strongly, creating a rhythm.

Pregnancy and after

Practise pelvic floor lifts through your pregnancy to keep the muscles of your pelvis, perineum and abdomen strong and elastic. Immediately after childbirth most women find they have too little sensation in the lower abdomen to be able to lift the pelvic floor. During the first postnatal weeks it is best to focus on breathing, the down-push on the floor, working the upper abdominal muscles, and visualization. Exercising from the outer, peripheral muscles inwards helps strengthen the stretched pelvic floor and this speeds the return of sensation.

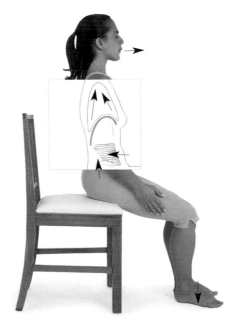

Strengthening the pelvic floor

Exercise can restore tone to a pelvic floor weakened by a sedentary lifestyle, illness or childbirth. As the muscles strengthen and return to their normal position in the pelvis, they balance muscles that interact with them. This improves body posture and bladder control, flattens the stomach, and may heighten sexual sensation. Above all, people who persevere with exercises to tone the pelvic floor say, when they succeed, that they just feel great.

To lift the pelvic floor, you have to squeeze the outer muscles between the tailbone and the front of the pelvis. Women find this easier than men because of the construction of their perineum (the bracing at the base of the pelvic floor, where the muscles you use to control the rectum and bladder are found). Internal lifting to exercise the pelvic floor is best known through the pioneering work of Dr. Arnold H. Kegel on the wellbeing of women during pregnancy. Women in many countries are taught his pelvic floor exercises as part of antenatal training.

At first, many women and most men find it hard to work out which muscles to try to move. This is not surprising. Not only are the pelvic floor muscles invisible, but they are beset by social taboos relating to elimination of wastes and to sexuality. But strong pelvic floor muscles bring such benefits to health and appearance that it is well worth persevering.

The male pelvic floor

Men can do pelvic floor exercises just as well as women. They can partially feel the lift through their own perineum – it is similar to the cold grip of what James Joyce in *Ulysses* called the 'scrotum-tightening sea'. Once they understand that it involves lifting the muscles they contract when they want to stop themselves from urinating, they move easily on to the next stage.

You can get a feel for which muscles to move by repeating the exercises on pages 130–31 over a few days, or by frequently stopping yourself urinating in mid-flow. Just using the pelvic floor muscles in this way strengthens them, causing them to feed back sensation.

Male pelvic floor seen from below

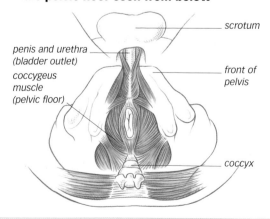

scrotum

penis and urethra (bladder outlet)

coccygeus muscle (pelvic floor)

front of pelvis

coccyx

Pelvic floor muscles

Stretching between the sitting bones, from the tailbone to the pubic bone at the front of the pelvis, thin sheets of muscle layered with connective tissue form a hammock. This is the pelvic floor. Its main function is to support the organs in the abdomen. The nervous system controls its inner layers, relaxing them to allow wastes to be eliminated from the body, or a baby to be born, while keeping the organs in place. When you cough and laugh, the outer muscles automatically contract to withstand the inner pressures, but you can also control them at will.

In men, the pelvic floor surrounds the anus and the penis. The coccygeus is the most important of the outer muscles in the diaphragm of pelvic floor muscles.

Pelvic floor lift

Once you have a feel for your pelvic floor muscles, you can move on to this exercise. Follow each pelvic floor lift with complete relaxation of all the muscles you have just squeezed. When you are used to these lifts, repeat 10 to 15 lifts in succession, 5 or 6 times a day. They are unnoticeable, so you can practise almost anywhere – in a train or on an aircraft, even while standing in a queue.

1 From the start position on page 130, push down both feet with equal pressure against the floor. This makes you sit higher and further back on the sitting bones. Then contract your buttock muscles, which lifts you off against the chair, and tighten the transversus abdominis muscles of the lower abdomen.

2 Breathing out to a slow count of six, lift the muscles between your tailbone and the front of your pelvis as high as you can. As your breath runs out, contract the outer muscles higher up in the abdomen. This lifts the pelvic floor higher, and as you squeeze the last of the air out, imagine your pelvic floor rising as high as your chest. Release, and with a very gentle down-push, relax your pelvic floor. Repeat this step four more times, taking a short in-breath between each repetition.

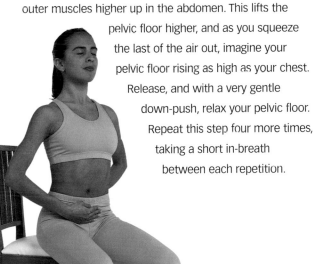

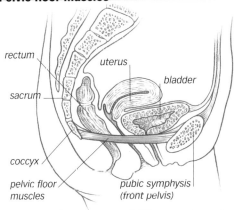

Pelvic floor muscles

rectum

uterus

bladder

sacrum

coccyx

pelvic floor muscles

pubic symphysis (front pelvis)

The pelvic floor muscles function best when the pelvis is upright and centered for gravity. When the pelvic floor is balanced and dynamically and structurally fit, as in the diagram above, the organs of the abdomen, which are connected to it, are in the middle of the pelvic space.

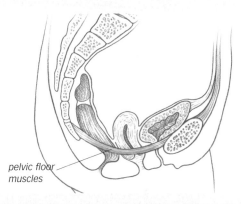

pelvic floor muscles

If the pelvic floor muscles are allowed to weaken and go slack, as in the diagram above, they can no longer support the abdominal organs, which sag and eventually prolapse or fall through the opening at the base of the pelvic girdle.

Breathing and lifting

As the pelvic floor contracts, the muscles that move the ribs also contract, preventing the chest from expanding, and the outer abdominal muscles tighten. The lower abdominals overlap the body's pivotal point between the hips and affect its centre of gravity. Holding the pelvic floor tightly contracted therefore restricts breathing, movement and speech, so it should be lifted briefly as a strengthening exercise and then relaxed.

The midpoint is deep in the pelvic floor. The diagrams on the right pinpoint its exact position. Clearly, being able to align the body in relation to its midpoint depends on the correct positioning of the pelvic floor.

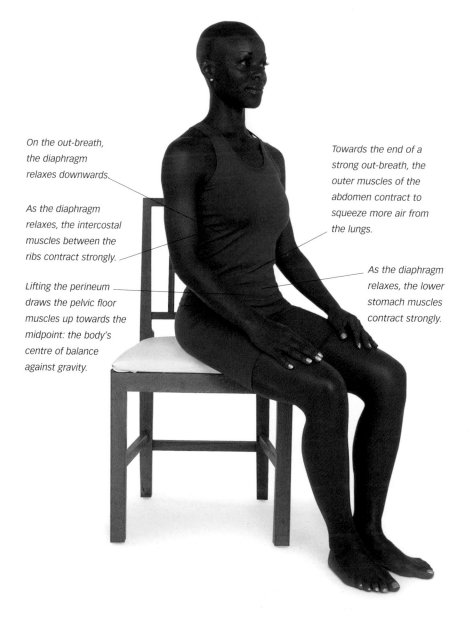

On the out-breath, the diaphragm relaxes downwards.

As the diaphragm relaxes, the intercostal muscles between the ribs contract strongly.

Lifting the perineum draws the pelvic floor muscles up towards the midpoint: the body's centre of balance against gravity.

Towards the end of a strong out-breath, the outer muscles of the abdomen contract to squeeze more air from the lungs.

As the diaphragm relaxes, the lower stomach muscles contract strongly.

Your body's central brace

The figure 8

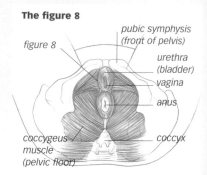

figure 8

pubic symphysis (front of pelvis)

urethra (bladder)

vagina

anus

coccygeus muscle (pelvic floor)

coccyx

Seen from below, the pelvic floor muscles make a figure 8 in the perineum. The loops are formed by the sphincter muscles around the anus and the sex organ and bladder. Men and women tighten and relax these muscles to prevent or allow wastes to pass out. Women can tighten the muscle that encircles the vagina. The corresponding muscle in men is involved in erection and ejaculation.

The perineum

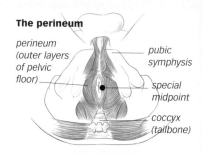

perineum (outer layers of pelvic floor)

pubic symphysis

special midpoint

coccyx (tailbone)

The perineum is the name for the diamond-shaped area between the pubic symphysis – the bone at the front of the pelvis – and the coccyx or tailbone. This illustration shows the location of the midpoint of the pelvis in the perineum. Purely for convenience, this book calls it the 'special midpoint'.

The special midpoint

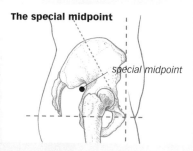

special midpoint

Man or woman, you should always carry a mental image of the location of your special midpoint. It lies just above the point where the anal canal passes through the perineum. Lifting it prevents strain when exercising or carrying something heavy.

The special midpoint

With its weight loaded on its centre or midpoint in the pelvic floor, the body counterbalances the force of gravity. However, some movements, such as holding a heavy object away from the body while lifting it, slouching when walking, or carrying a baby on the hip can make it lose its natural centre of balance. If they become habitual, these movements can affect the alignment of the spine. The exercises on the following pages will raise your awareness of the balancing role of the midpoint, and improve your posture and balance.

Although the body's midpoint can be located precisely, it cannot be felt, and no muscles move it. Like knowing where north is when travelling, it is, however, essential to carry a mental map on which your body's centre is marked, for your movements relate to it. The illustration on the right and the two diagrams opposite, on the left, pinpoint its exact position.

The special midpoint lift on page 137 helps align the body correctly in relation to its midpoint. This lift also directs the movements of the pelvic floor muscles towards the midpoint, which is why it is a useful exercise to know for when you are trying to lift heavy objects or to balance. Dancers, gymnasts and athletes can all benefit. It balances the trunk equally between the hip bones, lifts it out of the pelvis, and stabilizes it against gravity.

The strong pelvic floor lift shown on page 133 involves the outer muscles of the trunk, pelvis and thighs. The purpose of the special midpoint lift on page 137 is to direct these movements towards the midpoint. It is a much smaller movement – all you have to do is contract the muscles of the lower part of the pelvic floor, called the perineum. To distinguish between the pelvic floor lift, which raises the whole pelvic floor as high as possible, and the lower, less vigorous lifts described on the next two pages, I call lifting the perineum the 'special midpoint lift'.

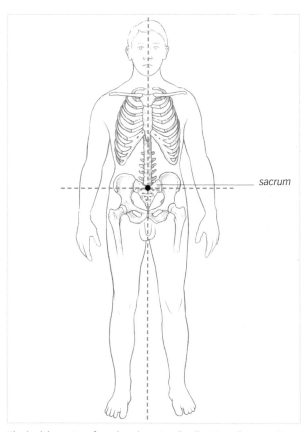

sacrum

The body's centre of gravity when standing lies 5 centimetres (2 inches) in front of the sacrum, at the level of the second of its five fused vertebrae. This is the midpoint – the spot where a horizontal line from hip to hip crosses a straight line drawn from head to feet through the exact centre of the body when standing.

Rhythmic lifting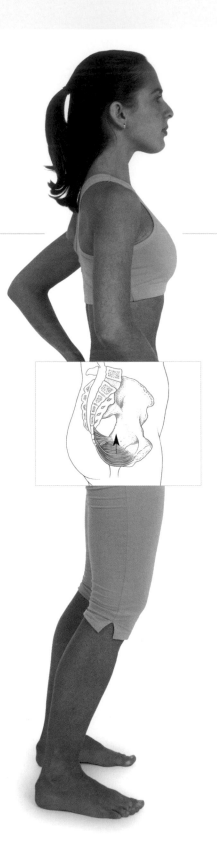

Lifting the special midpoint is a small movement, involving fewer muscles than lifting the pelvic floor, for instead of engaging the abdominal muscles, you contract the muscles under voluntary control in the lower part of the pelvic floor. Keep the muscles of the thighs, buttocks, abdomen and chest still, and move only those between the tailbone and the pubic bone at the front.

1 Stand, or sit on a chair in the start position on page 130. Take a short in-breath, and breathing out slowly to a count of six, lift only the outer muscles between the tailbone and the pubic bone. Relax, then repeat six times.

2 Keeping your breathing at the same speed, try to pull up faster while counting up to three, then let go. Repeat four times. While pulling up, do not involve the muscles of the buttocks or lower abdomen.
... breathe in ... and out ... and lift ... and two ... and three ... and release ...

3 Now try to lift on a count of one, and release on a count of one, breathing normally. Repeat many times, lifting and releasing to a regular rhythm.
breathing out ... lift ... release ... lift ... release ...

Special midpoint lift

The special midpoint lift involves lightly raising the voluntary muscles of the perineum. This pulls on the internal muscles of the pelvis, causing the tailbone to tuck further under and lengthening the end of the spine a little. Holding the back and front of the lower abdomen will help you feel the movement and the change in the angle of your pelvis to bring it more upright. This small movement transfers the balance of the spine from tail to head.

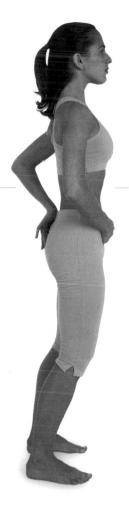

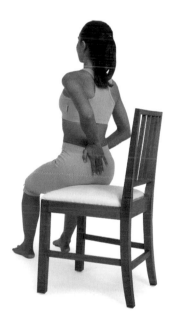

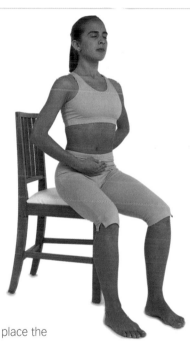

1 Adopt the start position on page 130, then place the index finger of your right hand on your tailbone, and cup your left hand against the muscles just above your pubic bone. Reverse the positions of your hands if you are left-handed. Take a short in-breath.

2 On a controlled out-breath do a few pelvic floor lifts, then push down equally with both feet and push the sitting bones against the chair. Close your eyes and imagine yourself urinating, then stopping in mid-flow, then practise the movement: hold and let go, hold again, for longer, and let go …and longer still…and let go. Spread the movement out from the pelvic floor and remember the effort you make.

3 Stand, keeping your hands on your tailbone and stomach, and bend your knees slightly. Breathe in, push down equally on both feet, and on a slow out-breath, repeat step 2. Repeat several times.

4 Now lift the midpoint and step forwards, then relax. Repeat until you can walk forwards, lifting and releasing. Finally, lift the special midpoint and take a few steps without releasing, then practise walking with the midpoint lifted.

Level 1 Review

The special midpoint lift necessarily changes the approach to the exercises, especially for the wall exercises. Level 1 therefore ends with a review of Stage 1 and Stage 2. Put aside some time every day or so to review a number of exercises, and refresh your experience by repeating them, bringing to them your new knowledge of the special midpoint lift. Review each exercise, then practise it with care and control. Use the special midpoint lift in every one, along with the equal down-push. Then move on to Level 2.

For pilates exercises to be effective regular practice is essential, and most people can manage a session two or three times a week only if they practise alone at home. Critical advice from a qualified teacher is equally important in order to perfect your technique, so try to get to a class, sign up for a course, or book a private session now and again.

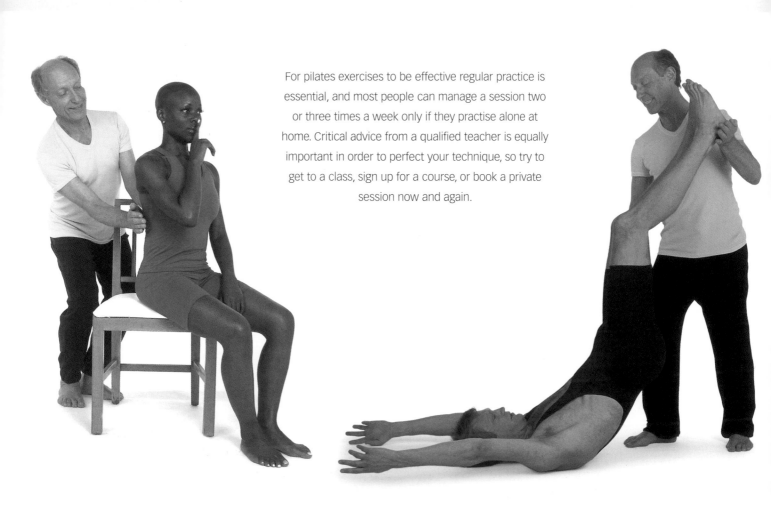

Return to level 1

Bear in mind that some of these exercises can be performed outside the practice room. The pelvic floor lifts can be practised anywhere – while travelling, for example, or sitting in a waiting room. Practise them when your energy level drops: getting the blood flow to the internal muscles going through contraction and release always helps. Exercises such as the triceps toner on page 108 and the foot rotations on pages 110–11 can relieve tension while working.

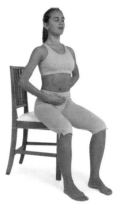

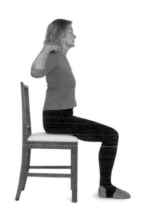

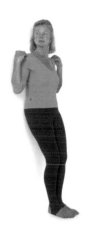

1 Do a series of 20 Pelvic floor lifts (see page 133): slow and hold… and fast and let go…slow and hold…and fast and let go…

2 Return to the Shoulder roll (see page 91) and repeat the equal down-push on the out-breath six times. Remember to add the special midpoint lift (see page 137).

3 Repeat the Back-to-the-wall owl head-swivel (see page 95) for the neck and upper back.

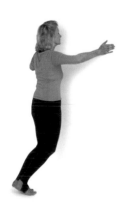

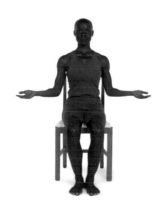

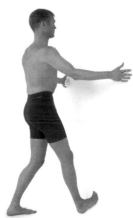

4 Now repeat the complete series of face-the-wall exercises to open the upper body, starting with the Upper back stretch on page 98 and finishing with the arm circles on pages 107–08…

5 Return to the Wake-up exercises to stretch the muscles of the lower abdomen, starting with Exercising the heart and lungs on page 126…

6 Finish by giving your legs a good workout, with the Calf stretch on page 114…

Level 2

As your body responds to regular practice the stretches and lifts you learned in Level 1 become easier and quicker, so that by this stage you can reprogram some of them into your warmup sequence for the beginning of each session. Level 2 focuses on integrating the movements you have learned so far into a balanced sequence of exercises to tone muscles and coordinate muscle groups. And while Level 1 focused mainly on the upper part of the body – the carriage of the head and neck, the balance of the torso, and the flexibility of the shoulders and upper chest – Level 2 concentrates on the hips and lower limbs.

Good habits of exercising and posture learned in earlier stages of the programme need to be carried forward into Level 2. Continue to practise three times a week, if not more often, and when possible start each practice session with a short period of self-massage (see pages 82–85), especially of the upper body. Practise the pelvic floor lift (see page 133) daily to maintain the strength of your internal abdominal muscles. And concentrate on raising awareness of your body's internal centre, bringing the special midpoint lift (see page 137) into every possible exercise. Always bear in mind that it is the focus of correct body posture, and that it protects the delicate internal structure of the abdomen, helping it withstand the intense pressures imposed on it by everyday activities. Never try to lift any heavy object without simultaneously lifting the special midpoint.

Achieving balance

A principal aim of Level 2 exercises is to balance the movements of the bilateral muscles attached to the pelvic girdle. An important function of this skeletal structure is to distribute the weight of the upper body to the legs and feet and so ensure the body's stability. It often happens, however, that a muscle on one side of the body is stiffer than its partner on the other side, sometimes because of an injury but often the result of a sedentary lifestyle. If the muscles of both thighs or both hips do not work symmetrically, the entire body will be unbalanced, affecting stance and movement. Level 2 exercises are designed to identify and loosen tight muscles in the lower back and in the hips and thighs, and strengthen the complex muscle structure of the knee and the ankle.

Breath control

From the first exercises in composure to the vigorous heart-lung stimulation on page 126, Level 1 explored the role of breathing in improving the effectiveness of exercising. Level 2 concentrates on breath control. Although breathing is governed by the central nervous system, which adapts respiratory depth and rhythm to maintain the balance of oxygen in the body with other gases, such as carbon dioxide, we exercise some control over the depth and rate of our breathing. Actors, singers, public speakers and wind instrument players learn to control their breathing in order to influence the timing, force, volume and quality of sounds they produce. Some dancers, gymnasts and athletes also use the breath to assist and punctuate their movements, and this same ability can improve the effectiveness of any exercise.

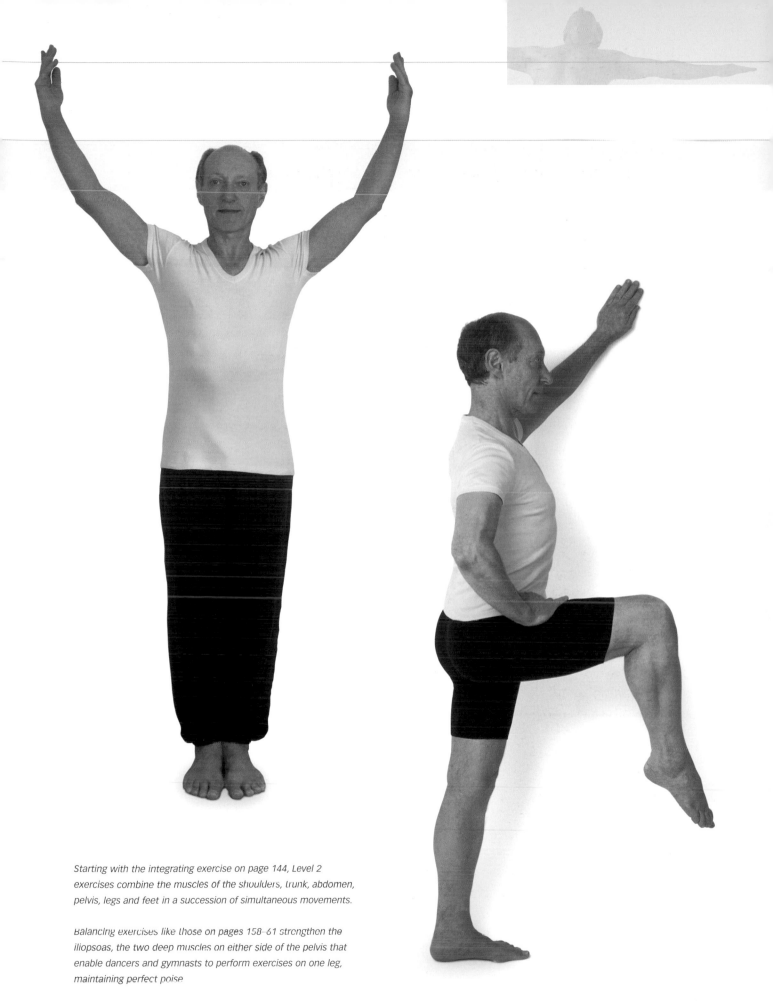

Starting with the integrating exercise on page 144, Level 2 exercises combine the muscles of the shoulders, trunk, abdomen, pelvis, legs and feet in a succession of simultaneous movements.

Balancing exercises like those on pages 158–61 strengthen the iliopsoas, the two deep muscles on either side of the pelvis that enable dancers and gymnasts to perform exercises on one leg, maintaining perfect poise.

Controlled breathing

Breathing helps you overcome blocks to physical expression caused by feelings and emotions. Anger and grief, even high excitement all affect breathing patterns, sometimes for prolonged periods. Fear makes us hold our breath, while living in a state of depression makes us tense up the muscles of the neck and shoulders and hold in the stomach and pelvic floor. The intercostal muscles that move the ribs are immobile, so breathing becomes rapid and shallow. The breathing exercises that begin Level 1 and Level 2 release tension and restore the breathing to its normal depth and rhythm, allowing rigid muscles to relax. With regular practice, breath control becomes second nature so that tension is defused before it can build up.

The breathing muscles

A thin sheet of muscle called the respiratory diaphragm works under the control of the brain to govern respiration, or breathing. You notice it when its natural rhythm is disturbed by hiccups. It is attached to the spine and the lower ribs.

Breathing in

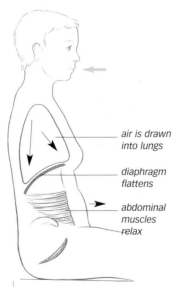

air is drawn into lungs

diaphragm flattens

abdominal muscles relax

Breathing out

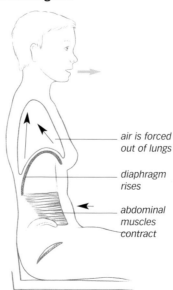

air is forced out of lungs

diaphragm rises

abdominal muscles contract

Breathing

We cannot control the action of the respiratory diaphragm, shown in the two illustrations on the left, but we have some control over the intercostal muscles in the spaces between the ribs.

When we inhale, *the respiratory diaphragm contracts and flattens (as illustrated far left). This creates a vacuum, and this draws air into the lungs. As they inflate, the rib cage expands to accommodate their greater volume. The intercostal muscles contract, raising the rib cage and breastbone up and out, increasing the volume of the chest. This draws more air into the lungs.*

When we exhale *the diaphragm relaxes into a dome shape (as the diagram on the left shows), the rib cage tightens, and the lungs deflate, expelling air. The intercostal muscles relax, closing the the rib cage and so compressing the lungs, forcing air out.*

Breath control

This exercise stretches the intercostal muscles that lift and lower the rib cage during breathing, encouraging you to use the full capacity of your lungs by controlling in-breaths as well as out-breaths. It can help recovery from the chesty cough that sometimes follows flu, and improve the breathing of anyone who has just stopped smoking, older people who experience shortness of breath when climbing stairs, and asthma sufferers.

1 Sit comfortably on an upright chair with your hands on your thighs. Breathe in through the nose and out through the mouth to a gentle rhythm until you reach an even measure of six slow counts in and six slow counts out. Feel your rib cage expand on the in-breaths, and slowly deflate on the out-breaths.

2 Continue to breathe out to a count of six, but place a forefinger on your lips to hinder the outflow of air, as if you were trying to inflate a balloon through pursed lips. As each out-breath ends, practise the special midpoint lift.

3 Take a short in-breath, breathing in only as much air as you need for another long, forced out-breath, and repeat five more times. Now purse your lips as you take a long, slow in-breath, and breathe out more rapidly. Feel your back and ribs open and widen. Repeat until you reach an even rhythm.

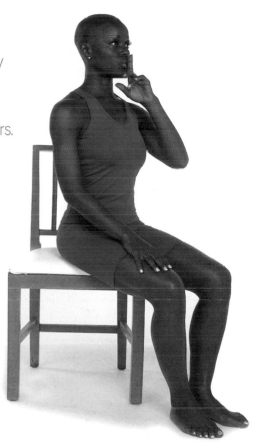

Resisted in-breaths

Stress combined with lack of exercise encourages a tendency to overuse the upper lungs and underuse the diaphragm, resulting in fast, shallow breathing. Level 1 exercises on pages 88–89 focus on slow, controlled out-breaths to relax the muscles used in breathing. Level 2 exercises work on controlled in-breaths and on deep breathing.

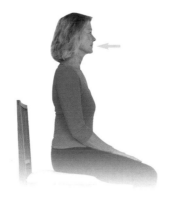

If you find it hard to take long, slow in-breaths, visualization can help you learn. When trying to force or slow the in-breath, some people experience a panicky feeling, as if they are not getting enough air. This is a normal reflex. Gently persuade yourself to override it and regain control of your breathing by imagining that your lungs are a balloon you are slowly filling with air.

Dynamic stances

While working through Level 1 you stretched all parts of your body, from head to toe, and you stretched and loosened many muscles. The movements on this page take you one step forward to a point from which you can begin to work towards integration – the coordination of the movements of several groups of muscles. For example, the arm circles in Level 1 used all the muscles of the shoulder, whereas the arm movements on these pages combine movements of the shoulders, trunk, abdomen, pelvis, legs and feet in a series of simultaneous movements. Integrated movements look and feel smoother and more coordinated and controlled.

Integrating exercise

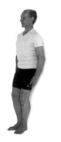

Start position
Stand with your back to the wall, about 30 centimetres (12 es) away, your arms by your sides, and your feet almost parallel, then lean back against the wall so that your lower back and shoulders rest on it.

This stance is a variation of the Arm circle, palms away on page 108. For that exercise you faced the wall, but here you have your back to the wall, and this makes it more difficult to keep your arms close to the wall as you circle them. It is also harder to work the upper body. Persevere with trying to touch the wall with your hands as they slide up, and stretch your chest quite hard. Visualize the stance and movements before attempting them.

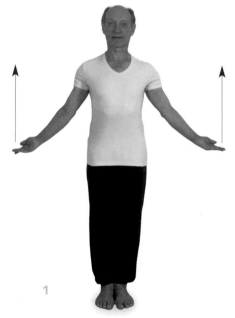

1

1 From the start position, press your heels together, and bend your knees. Stretch your neck up, hold your head upright so it does not touch the wall, and look straight ahead. Take a long, slow out-breath, and open your hands and forearms out to the sides, keeping them close to the wall and turning the palms up.

2 On the same slow out-breath, and keeping your hands close to the wall, begin circling your arms upwards. When your arms reach shoulder height, push down against the floor to stretch the upper body up from the special midpoint. At the same time, relax and stretch your upper back to allow the shoulder blades to swivel open, easing the path of your arms as you circle them above your head.

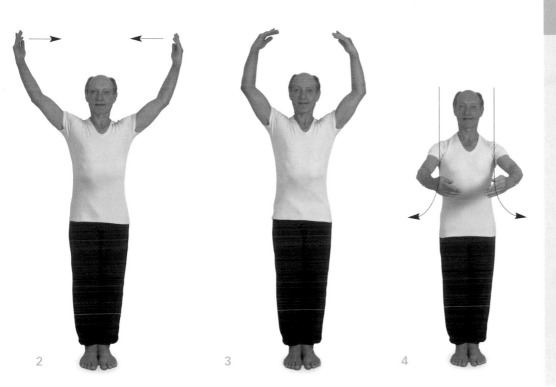

2　　　　　　　　3　　　　　　　　4

Points to watch

- Do not press your head back against the wall, since this tightens the muscles of the neck and shoulders.
- The feet are active, so that when you push down they rebound against the floor, giving a small upward push.
- Keep your shoulders back and your shoulder blades pressing against the wall, especially in step 3.
- Hold the special midpoint lift throughout.
- Keep your buttock muscles relaxed.

3 Open your shoulders and slowly begin to lower your arms to the front, reaching forward as you do so. Keep your shoulder blades back and square against the wall, and your forearms parallel.

4 Bring your hands down as far as your waist, then down beside your thighs, and rest briefly. Then take a short in-breath, and on a long, slow out-breath, push both feet down against the floor, lift from the special midpoint, and repeat steps 1–4.

5 Take a short in-breath and turn your hands back so the palms face out and your thumbs touch the wall. Keeping your shoulder blades pressing against the wall, circle your arms on a slow out-breath, as in steps 2–4. Relax your shoulders down and outward as your arms reach shoulder height, and rotate your arms a little as they rise above your head to keep the palms facing out, then bring your arms forward and lower them. Repeat step 5 four times.

Rest and repeat

Relax, step forward and walk around for a moment to clear your mind. Resume the start position and repeat steps 1–5 four times, breathing evenly throughout, then rest.

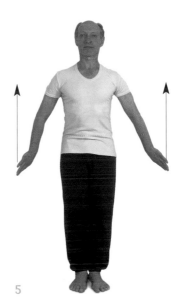

5

Navel-to-spine

Some people are taught to exercise the abdominal muscles by pulling the navel back towards the spine and tucking the pelvis under to flatten the lumbar spine. Try this out, and you find that pulling the abdominal muscles in makes you tighten your rib cage. This restricts free movement of the respiratory diaphragm and the lungs. If, as some teachers advise, this movement is practised frequently over a long period it not only interferes with breathing but also encourages defective posture and inhibits normal movement and self-expression.

I am in accord with teachers of the Alexander Technique, who avoid this movement in their teaching. I advise substituting other abdominal exercises from the repertoire. The abdominal wake-up calls on pages 126–28, if practised every two or three days, will effectively tighten slack abdominal muscles without exerting pressure on the abdominal organs and without restricting breathing.

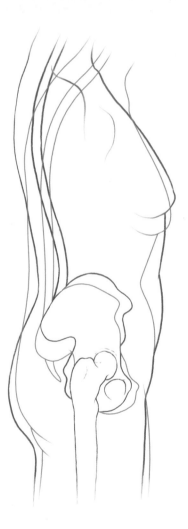

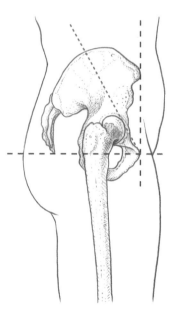

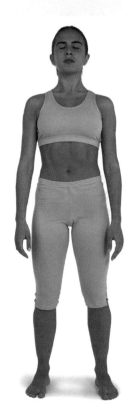

The special midpoint lift in Level 1 has the effect of maintaining the pelvic tilt at the correct angle to the horizontal, illustrated on the left. The tightened muscles of the pelvic floor exert a pull on the muscles of the lower abdomen in front and on the coccyx behind. This action improves posture and balance without restricting respiration.

The action of pulling the navel towards the spine, taught in many pilates classes, interferes with breathing by constricting the ribs. This movement, if practised daily over a prolonged period, can flatten the lumbar spine, which has the effect of straightening out all of the spine's natural curves and depressing the tailbone. In time, the back loses its flexibility. Eventually, distorted posture and inhibited movement become a feature of the body. I have replaced navel-to-spine in my exercises with the special midpoint lift described on page 137.

Stability and balance

The weight of the upper body is channelled down the spine and around the pelvic girdle, which transmits it via the hip joints to the legs and feet. The pelvic girdle encircles the body's centre of gravity, so its position and balance are important in maintaining stability. To be able to do this effectively, your pelvis needs to be stable and upright, and for this it relies on secure ligaments and elastic tendons and muscles in the hips and thighs. These balance the movements of your spine and torso, hips, and lower limbs. An essential part of your exercise programme is therefore to work on the stability and flexibility of your pelvis, legs, and feet.

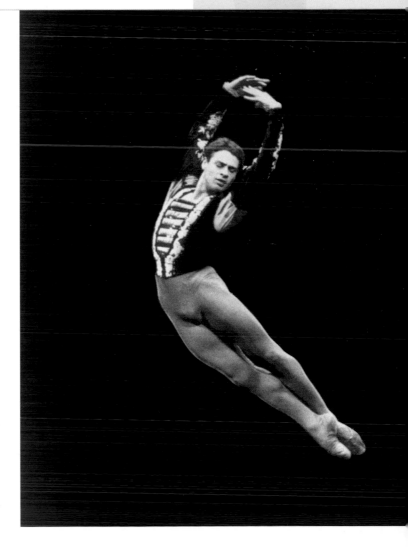

In a healthy body, some muscles work together and others in opposition to keep the body functioning and agile. Anyone who has experienced lower back pain, a stiff hip, or sciatic nerve pain in the buttock and leg can describe the lopsided feeling these conditions produced. Each muscle has specific functions, and when weakened, tight, or affected by injury or misuse, it will have a negative influence on overall balance and structural fitness.

To maintain the correct structural alignment throughout the body, it is therefore essential to maintain the strength and elasticity of these muscles. The smallest misalignment can have a bad effect on posture, and this will take its toll in wear and tear on some body part. Physiotherapists, osteopaths, and others are trained to rebalance the affected structures to aid recovery. These Level 2 exercises can help correct minor stiffness and problems, but if practised regularly, they help prevent misalignments and malfunctions.

The exercises in the next pages are the easiest and most practical for working on the muscles and tendons of the lower body from hips to feet, to strengthen them and keep them flexible and balanced. Overall fitness radiates from the pelvic area, and for those people whose working lives reduce their mobility to little more than sitting and standing, they are essential to maintain flexibility and mobility.

All the muscle structures of the body are contributing to the execution of this leap. The position of the head in relation to the torso indicates that the dancer has perfect control over the direction of the movement.

Sock stretch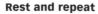

This exercise introduces the hip stretches and rolls on the following pages. It eases the hips and loosens the lower back. I designed it for a client over 90 years old who was beginning to find it difficult to put his socks on in the mornings, hence the name. It is surprising how many people, decades younger, find one hip much stiffer than the other, perhaps because of the way they habitually sit or because of an injury that happened a while ago.

Warning

The sock stretch is not for anyone who has had a hip replacement. If your hips feel rather stiff and need easing to make them more mobile, practise the sock stretch regularly, but always go gently. Do not force the stretch.

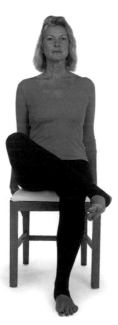
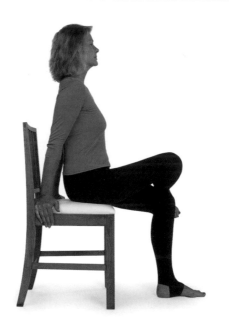
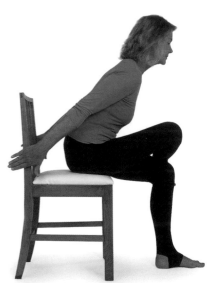

1 Sit on an upright chair, feet together, and press both feet on the floor. Lift your head and spine, and sit up on the sitting bones. Slide your right foot up along your shin. Supporting your right knee with your hand if necessary, raise your foot farther up until it rests on your left knee.

2 Ease your right foot into place and, still stretching up from the sitting bones, breathe in, and breathe out slowly for a count of six.

3 Lean forward to increase the stretch around the right hip, take a short in-breath, and hold while breathing out slowly to a count of six.

4 Breathe in, then repeat step 3, curving forward as far as you can.

Rest and repeat

Relax and bring the right foot down to the floor, then release the left foot and slide it up against the right shin. Repeat steps 1–4, then get up and walk around.

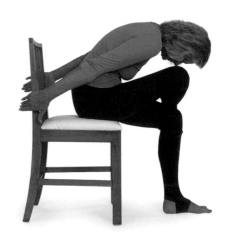

Exercising the lateral hip rotators

Beneath the buttock muscles is a group of six muscles that link the sacrum, the tissues surrounding the sitting bones, the hip joints, and the heads of the thigh bones (see page 54). They rotate the hips and thighs outwards. The balance of these muscles can affect the sciatic nerve, causing pain if they are not aligned. They tend to shorten, restricting movement, and need to be stretched to even out their balance. This exercise works on these deep muscles.

1 Lie on your left side with your knees bent and in line with your hips and shoulders. Place a towel or a supporting cushion or foam pad underneath your head and neck.

2 Press the sides of your feet together, then turn the right thigh outwards, pivoting on the hip joint and foot. The knee lifts and opens to the side. Hold for about 30 seconds, return the knee to its start position, and repeat four times.

Repeat and rest
Now lie on your right side, and repeat step 2 five times, lifting the left knee.

The pivoting hip
Try to keep the hip still and move only the knee. Think of the hip at the top as a pivot. The leg is attached to it, but moves freely, like a pendulum.

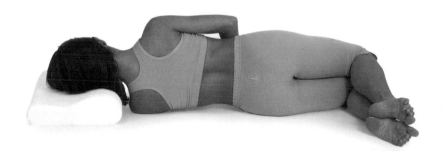

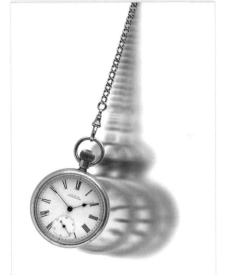

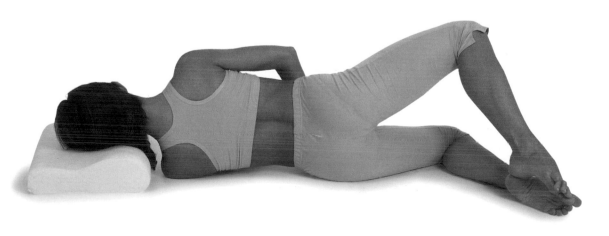

Hip rolls

The three exercises that follow work the muscles of the lower back and the buttocks. They need to be carried out in sequence. If, when you begin the hip roll stretch on this page, you find that either hip is stiff, massage it with a stick or a ball (see pages 86–87) to ease the gluteus maximus in the upper part of the pelvis. Then try the hip roll stretch again, and if your hip is easier, move on to the stretches on pages 152–53. You may find that you feel more of a stretch on one side of the body, or in one hip, but continue to exercise both hips, and do not reduce the time you spend on either side. Whenever one knee is stretched over sideways, try to relax and let the weight of the leg increase the stretch.

Hip roll stretch

A stretch to loosen the lower back muscles, the quadratus lumborum, and other muscles that connect the pelvis, ribs and spine at the waist, plus the gluteal muscles of the buttocks.

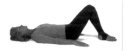

Start position
Lie on a mat on your back with your knees bent. Rest your head on a support cushion, a folded towel, or a thin book to stretch your neck and position it in line with the spine. Your arms should be close to your sides, hands level with hips.

1 From the start position stretch your arms above your head, bend your knees, move your heels together, and press both feet down against the floor. Now slide your right heel up your left leg until it almost reaches the knee. Press the inside of it against the inside of the knee. Breathe in.

2 On a slow out-breath and keeping your ankle pressing against your knee, roll your two legs over to the left until your left knee almost touches the floor. Keep your shoulders down, and turn your head to face right. Hold for 30 seconds, then return to the step 1 position. Repeat three times.

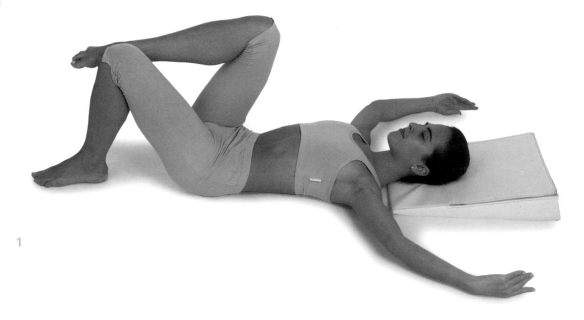

1

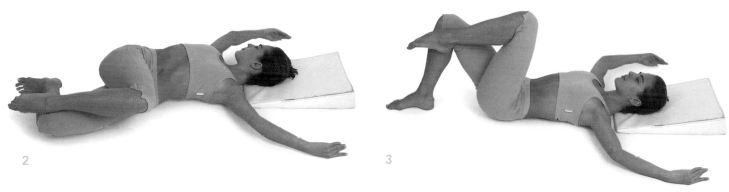

2

3

3 Return to the start position and rest, then slide your left heel up your right leg almost to the knee, pressing the inside of the heel against the inside of your left knee.

4 Repeat step 2, this time rolling both legs over to the right side. Hold for about 30 seconds, relaxing your left hip and feeling the stretch, then relax. Repeat three times.

4

Repeat and rest
Repeat steps 1–4 four times, then stretch your legs out, return your arms and hands to your sides, and rest.

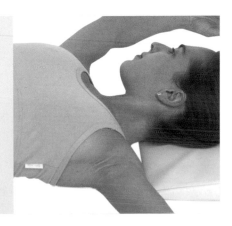

Positioning the shoulders
As you raise your arms above your head in step 1, pull down the lats and pecs to keep your shoulders down. When you roll your legs to the left and then to the right in steps 2–4, keep both shoulders touching the floor throughout.

Hip rotations

This variation on the Sock stretch on page 150, carried out while lying on the floor instead of sitting in a chair, stretches the piriformis, one of the hip rotator muscles (see page 54). When this muscle is tight, it traps the sciatic nerve, causing pain. Keep both shoulders touching the mat as you roll your legs over.

1 From the start position on page 150, stretch your arms above your head and move your heels close to your buttocks. Raise your right foot and rest the ankle on your left knee, easing it into place. Press your right foot down against the outside of your left knee and press the right knee downward, trying to rest it at a right angle from the body, then dorsiflex the right foot (bend it upward).

2 On a slow out-breath, and treating the two legs as a unit, roll them over to the left and turn your head to the right. Hold for about 30 seconds, consciously relaxing the hips to stretch the rotator muscles and the right buttock.

3 Keeping your legs in the same position, lift them into their position in step 1, then repeat step 2 rolling them over to the left again. Repeat twice more: lift the legs, and roll to the left; lift, and roll.

4 Lift the legs as a unit once more, and when they are in the step 2 position, release your right foot and place it on the floor. Then repeat step 1, this time resting your left ankle on your right knee.

5 On an out-breath, roll both legs as a unit over to the right, turning your head to the left. Hold, relaxing the hip muscles and stretching the left buttock, then repeat step 4, lifting the legs, and rolling to the right, lifting and rolling to the right. Finally, lift again, release the left foot, and replace it on the floor.

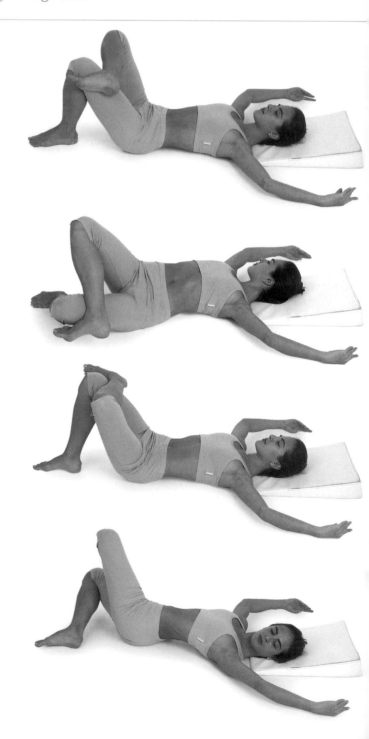

The crossed-knees hip-rotator stretch

The sequence of three exercises ends with this tough stretch, which extends the effects of the hip stretch opposite to the hip rotators and the gluteals.

1 From the start position on page 150, move your heels in toward your buttocks, and cross your right knee over your left knee, dropping the right foot close to the outside of the left foot.

2 Treating your two bent legs as a unit, roll them over to the left. Hold for about 30 seconds, allowing the weight of the right thigh to stretch and the deep rotator muscles of the right hip and the right buttock muscle.

3 Keeping your knees crossed, slowly raise them and move them over to the right, now allowing the weight of the right knee to stretch the tensor fasciae latae muscle and the iliotibial tract in the left thigh. Hold for at least 30 seconds, and relax.

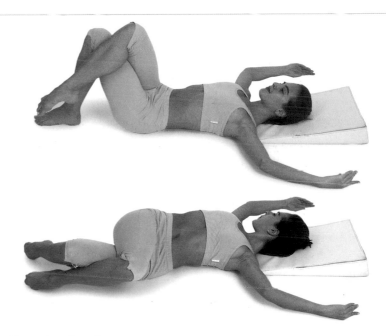

Repeat and rest

Repeat steps 2 and 3 three times. Then, slowly raise your legs to the step 1 position, and release your left leg into the start position. Repeat steps 1–3 three times on each side, with your left knee crossed over your right knee. To finish, stretch both legs and relax.

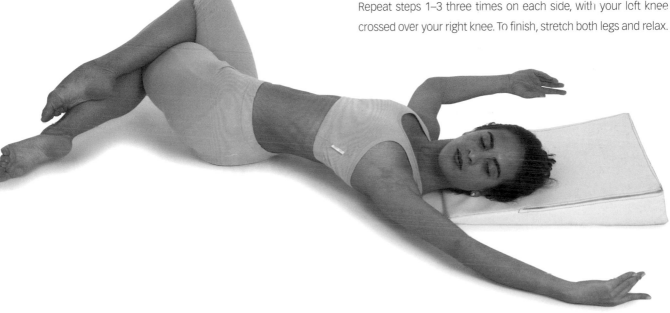

Working the multifidus ⇨

Several Level 2 exercises gently stretch the deep multifidus muscles of the spine. These muscles can be overstretched by vigorous exercising, so this exercise must not be practised hard or in isolation. It is included specifically to help anyone with lower back pain that an osteopath has identified as stemming from a multifidus problem. Before you attempt it, you must have worked through the hip and thigh exercises in Level 1 (see pages 115–22), and it must only be done at the end of the sequence of Level 2 exercises beginning with the hip rolls on pages 150–51. Do no more than four repeats on each side to start, working up, in time, to six. This exercise also works the transversus abdominis, which supports the lower back.

Warning
Do this exercise only after consulting your physician, and only as the last exercise in the sequence beginning on pages 150–51. Never practise it by itself. Doing so could tighten one side of the spine more than the other.

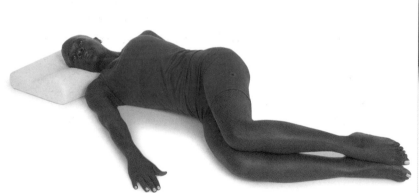

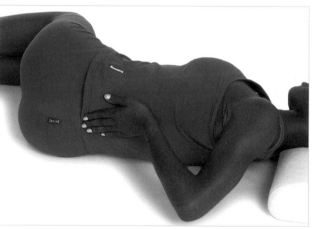

1 Lie on your right side and rest your head on a support cushion, a folded towel, or a thin book. Press the insides of your feet together, bring your knees together so they touch, bend them, and slide them up until your heels are in line with your spine. Stretch your right arm out, and turn the palm down, pointing the hand towards your knees.

2 Press your left hand on your lower back where your spine and pelvis join to feel your lower back rotate as you go on to lift your knees in step 3.

3 Apply the special midpoint lift, and press your knees together and your feet against the floor. Pressing your right arm down against the floor for resistance, and swivelling the lower half of your body against your trunk, swing your knees upwards, then return to the step 1 position. Repeat three or four times, then rest.

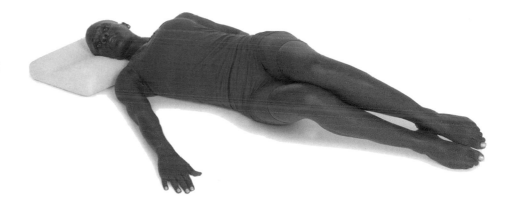

Repeat and rest

Repeat steps 1–3 lying on your left side with your left arm stretched out and using your right hand to feel your lumbar spine swivel.

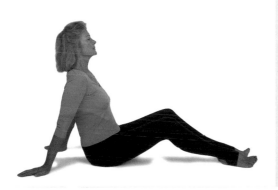

Aches in the lower back

A severe jolt or injury often causes problems with the multifidus muscles. Less severe lower back problems resulting from bad posture, a jerk when standing up or an invertebral disk problem, require different exercises. Practise the pelvic floor lift on page 133, then the abdominal muscle wake-ups on pages 126–28, and progress to the hip rotations on pages 152–53. Gently practise this sequence of exercises every day, and your back will quickly strengthen and the pain and stiffness will ease and disappear. Use deep massage with a tennis ball below the hip bone at the back (see page 87). Always check a lower back problem with your physician before exercising.

The multifidus

The multifidus consists of a number of small muscles that scale the spine on either side from the sacrum to the neck. Other deep muscles of the spine lie alongside, and each connects a pair or a group of vertebrae. If any muscle in the multifidus group is slack, there is instability in rotating, flexing and stretching the spine, so the multifidus is the key to the balanced function of the lower back muscles.

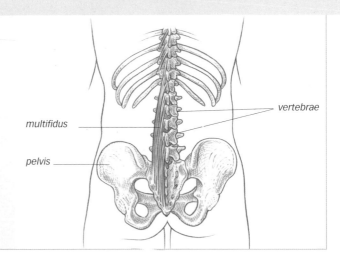

vertebrae

multifidus

pelvis

Balancing the iliopsoas

The iliopsoas forms a bridge between trunk and legs and is the main muscle that flexes, or bends, the hip. It has a major role in balancing the deep abdominal muscles that keep the pelvis at the correct tilt and level at the hips. If the iliopsoas tightens or loosens, this symmetry is destroyed, resulting, in time, in a deepened lumbar curve and a pot belly. The iliopsoas (usually simplified to 'the psoas' responds to the hip flexor stretches on pages 116–17. These will stretch a taut psoas and strengthen one that has been weakened, perhaps through lack of exercise, and in time it will restore the internal stabilizing balance of the pelvis. Begin with the strengthening exercise below, and go on to the variation, then to Precision balancing on page 158.

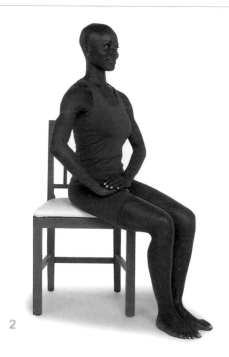

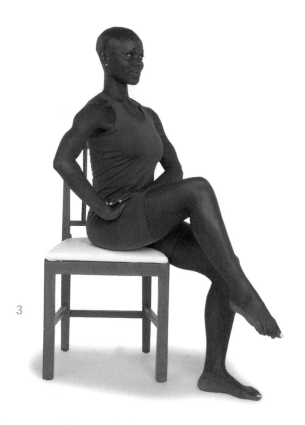

1 Sit on a high-backed chair with your hands on your thighs and your feet together. Push both feet with equal pressure down against the floor, and pull yourself up on to the sitting bones.

2 Put one hand on the other, and insert the joined hands into the right side of your groin.

3 Keeping your left foot pushing down against the floor, lift your right leg, and as you do so, press your hands down to resist the lift. Now, take a short in-breath and, breathing out

for a count of six, sustain the push, while sitting tall and upright and lifting from the midpoint and from the sitting bones.

Repeat and rest

Repeat steps 2 and 3 twice, then relax. When you are ready, repeat steps 1–3, inserting your joined hands between the left thigh and hip, and lifting your left leg. Then walk around to stretch your legs.

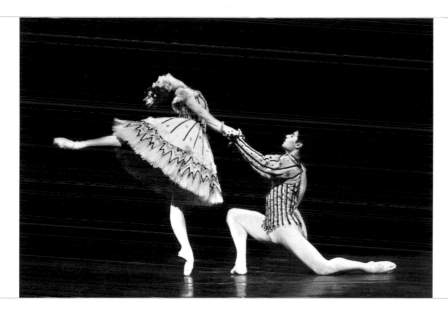

In this beautiful pose the dancer uses the hip flexors and the adductors of the leg on which she is standing to stabilize the leg at the supporting hip. This enables her to abduct (raise) the other leg 90° from the horizontal to as high as 180°.

Variation

This more demanding exercise balances the body in a sitting position, strengthening not only the hip flexors but also the body structures that pull the shoulders down.

Sit as in step 1, then raise your left hand, palm facing inwards above your head and lift your right knee. Insert your right hand in the fold between thigh and hip, and use it to resist the lift of the knee. Repeat four times on an out-breath to a count of six, then repeat, lifting the left knee. Remember to sit tall and upright during the push and to counter-press against the floor with the opposite foot throughout.

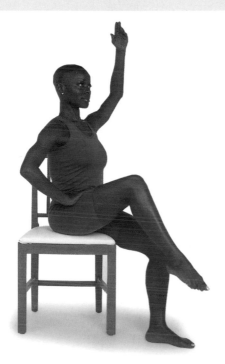

Strengthen the weak side

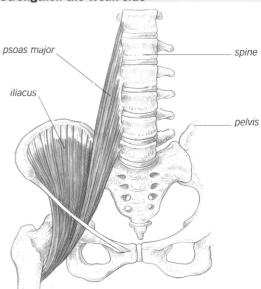

psoas major

spine

iliacus

pelvis

The iliopsoas consists of a pair of muscles, the iliacus and the psoas major, on either side of the body (see page 55). If you resist the push with the hands in this balancing exercise more effectively with one leg than with the other, the psoas on the weaker side may need strengthening. Start on the weak side and end with an extra repetition on that side. Once both sides resist the push evenly, do equal numbers of repetitions. After you finish, stand and walk around.

Precision balancing

The psoas is central to achieving balance. When a dancer stands on one leg with the trunk centrally positioned over the hip joint and aligned with the foot, the psoas is hard at work with the adductors – the muscles that move the thigh inwards – and the buttock and hip muscles. Try this exercise when you are confident that the psoas muscles on both sides of your body are equally strong. Then practise the following steps as often as you can.

1 Stand facing a wall with your feet together, turn right, and rest your left hand on the wall for support. Place your right hand lightly at the junction between your right hip and thigh. Lifting from the midpoint, push down with equal pressure on both feet as if you were standing on a springboard, preparing to dive. (Your feet and ankles have enough spring to enable you to push off from a flat floor.)

2 Lift your right knee in front so you balance on your left leg. Push your left foot down, stretch your left leg, engaging the hip flexors at the front of the thigh, and lift from the midpoint to stand tall. Do not drop your right knee – picture yourself pointing your right thigh from your buttock. Hold for six slow out-breaths, then lower your foot and rest.

3 Turn to face the opposite direction and repeat step 1, resting your right hand against the wall. Push down on both feet with equal pressure, release your left leg, and lift the knee up in front. Push down hard on the right foot and stretch from heel to hip to balance, steadying yourself against the wall if necessary. Hold for six slow out-breaths, keeping your left knee high, then lower your foot and rest.

Rest and repeat

Repeat steps 1–3 three times, balancing first on the right leg, then on the left, each time on a slow out-breath.

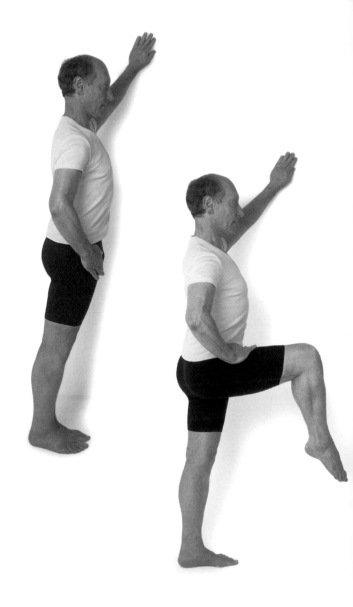

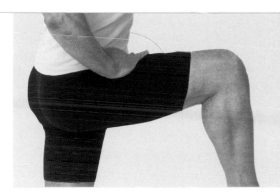

Variation: Free balancing

Repeat steps 1 and 2, this time pressing down on your right hand and pushing upward with your right knee in step 2. Hold still for a slow out-breath, keeping your hips aligned horizontally as you push down into the fold between thigh and hip to resist the upward pressure from your thigh. Still breathing out, push your left foot hard against the floor, feeling your left leg and hip straighten. Stretch up and relax your shoulders. Breathe in, and on a slow out-breath, lift your hand from the wall and balance freely. Lower your right foot and rest. Turn and repeat, lifting your left knee. Repeat the variation three times.

Key balance ⇨

This is a key exercise to balance the psoas and all the surrounding structures of the pelvis. It feeds into the central balance at the inner ear, strengthening and reinforcing your natural sense of balance.

1 Repeat steps 1 and 2 of the Precision balancing exercise opposite. Keeping your right knee lifted high, your hips level, and your left hand pressing against the wall for support, close your eyes so that you balance from the midpoint without the help of your eyesight. At first this feels quite insecure, but it feels easier with practice. Hold for a slow count of six, and rest.

2 Turn to face the opposite direction and repeat step 1 with your eyes closed, balancing on your right leg and lifting your left knee. Repeat two or three times.

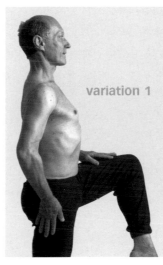

variation 1

Variation 1

Repeat the exercise, and when you feel secure lift your hand from the wall, rest it on your thigh, and balance freely. Pressing the other hand down between hip and thigh steadies your balance.

Variation 2

Once you have achieved steadier balance, repeat the exercise, lifting the opposite arm up above the head as one leg and foot take your weight.

Achieving balance

When you raise your knee in both exercises and their variations, steady yourself by resting one hand lightly on the wall or against a door frame. You will find it easier to balance if your weight is centred from the midpoint on the ball and toes of the foot you are standing on, and if you push the heel down strongly. As you do so, feel the stretch along the front of the hip and thigh.

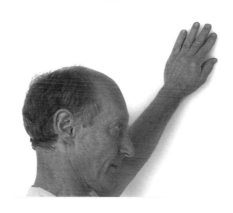

Strengthening the quads

Although they are not involved in bending the knee, the tendons of all four quads – the large, four-headed muscle stretching from the knee to the hip – are attached to the kneecap. When the knee is stretched and bent, they tighten and relax, pulling the kneecap up and down and extending the lower leg. Weak quads, especially a weak vastus medialis, may cause the kneecap to fail to find its correct position when the knee is straightened (see page 123). The knee bends and heel rises on page 113 stretch and strengthen the quads. This exercise tests their strength and tones them.

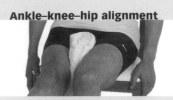

Ankle–knee–hip alignment

If you cannot feel the vastus medialis, make a fist, or roll up a towel or a magazine, and place it between your knees. This aligns your leg from ankle to hip, which tightens the vastus medialis so you can feel it. Women may need to use something larger – a folded bath towel or telephone book.

1 Sit on the edge of a straight-backed chair with your knees and feet touching and pointing forward. Press your feet down to lift on to the sitting bones, and sit upright. Now stretch out your right leg to straighten the knee, and place one hand on the thigh just above the hollow on the inside by the kneecap. You should be able to feel whether the vastus medialis, beneath your hand, is strong and hard. Press your knees together to make it work.

2 Lower your right foot to the floor, then take a short in-breath and straighten your right knee again, turning your right foot inwards as you lift your right leg. Hold for six slow counts, while checking the muscle. You should find it has tightened as you lifted your leg. Then rest the foot on the ground briefly. Repeat six times.

Repeat and rest

Repeat steps 1 and 2, this time lifting your left leg and turning your left foot inwards on each lift, and feeling the inside of the knee with one hand to check what has happened to the muscle.

Variation

Sit as in step 1, and stretch out your right leg, heel touching the floor, toes dorsiflexed. Take a short in-breath, and on a slow out-breath, push down on your right heel and tighten your quads from knee to hip. Rest and repeat six times, then repeat the exercise, stretching out your left leg and tightening the muscles.

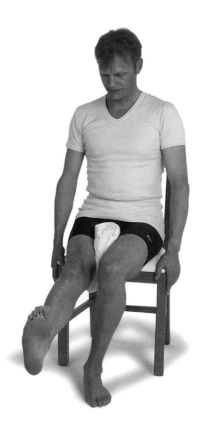

Strengthening the vastus medialis

This alternative exercise tones and strengthens the adductor muscles of the hips and thighs (which move the leg in toward the body). Because you do it lying down, it is more difficult than the knee bends on page 113. In steps 2 and 3, you should feel the inner thigh muscles working, especially the vastus medialis, one of the four quadriceps muscles.

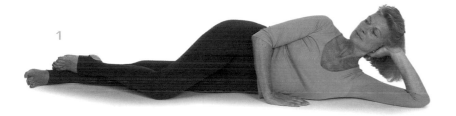

1 Lie on a mat on your left side with your left leg extended underneath. Rest your head on your left hand or on a thin cushion.

2 Bend your right leg and move the foot left to rest it on the floor in front of the left knee. Lift your extended left leg off the floor and dorsiflex the foot (turn the toes up towards you). Take a short in-breath and hold your left leg up for six slow counts, then rest it on the ground briefly. Repeat this step six times.

3 Now repeat the exercise lying on your right side and lifting your right leg.

Repeat and rest

Repeat steps 1–3 six times, then rest briefly before getting up and walking around briefly.

The vastus medialis

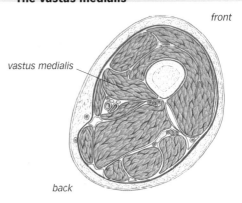

front

vastus medialis

back

This diagram is a cross-section through the right thigh, showing the four heads of the quadriceps muscle, of which the vastus medialis is the one running down the inside of the thigh. Most of the vastus medialis is deep inside the thigh, but it forms a bulge just above the knee.

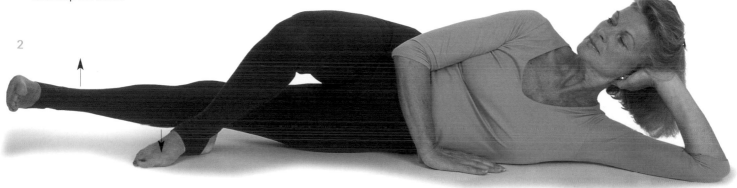

Working the adductors

The five adductors inside the thigh move the legs towards the midline of the body. You use them to cross one thigh over the other. These muscles are often under-exercised and become soft and weak, making the inside of the thigh flabby. Three exercises on pages 122–24 stretch and pull them, and this one strengthens them. Keep your shoulders open, your lats down, and look straight ahead.

1 Sit on the edge of an upright chair, push both feet against the floor with equal pressure, and place your hands on the insides of your thighs.

2 Take a short in-breath, and on a slow out-breath and to a count of six, press inwards with your thighs and push your hands outwards to meet the pressure equally. Repeat six times.

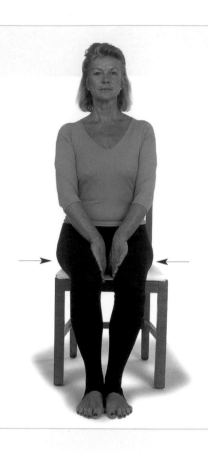

Working the abductors

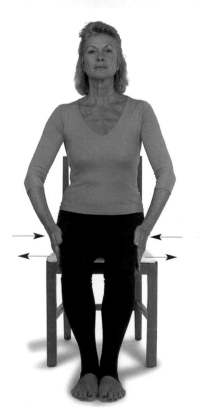

The abductors, which move the thighs outwards, include the tensor fasciae latae and the gluteal muscles of the buttocks. The exercises on pages 122–24 stretch them; this one tones and strengthens them. Keep your shoulders open, your lats down, and look straight ahead.

1 Sit on the edge of an upright chair, push both feet against he floor with equal pressure, and place your hands on the outsides of your thighs.

2 On a slow out-breath, press outwards with your thighs and push your hands inwards to meet the pressure equally. Repeat six times.

Buttocks and thighs

The exercises on the next seven pages work all the large muscle groups of the lower body: the gluteal muscles of the buttocks and the muscles that move and rotate the hips and thighs. Concentrate on these exercises if you want to tighten and streamline your seat and thighs. These exercises also strengthen the hamstrings, which contribute to maintaining the pelvic tilt, and balance the quads.

Stretch and tighten

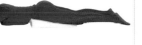

Start position
Lie on the floor on your front, with a folded towel or a cushion under your stomach to support the lower back. Your feet are parallel and pointed, the insteps touching the mat. Bend your elbows, place your hands palms down, fingertips on the mat level with your head. Pull down your lats and align your neck with your spine.

Here is a simple way of working the buttocks and hamstrings. Remember to breathe out as you stretch out your legs.

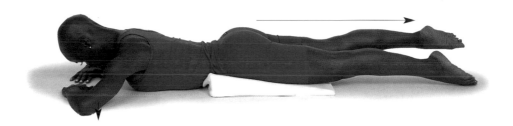

1 Breathe in and push your forearms down against the floor while lifting internally from the special midpoint, so the transversus abdominis muscles in the lower abdomen pull up, away from the floor. On the out-breath, push both feet down against the floor,

extend upwards from the waist, and stretch both legs away from the hips and toward your feet.

2 On a slow out-breath, raise your left leg and foot off the mat, stretching the leg along its length from

the sitting bones to the heel. Hold for six counts. Repeat six times.

Repeat and rest
Repeat steps 1 and 2, raising the right leg in step 2, rest briefly, then repeat three more times, and rest.

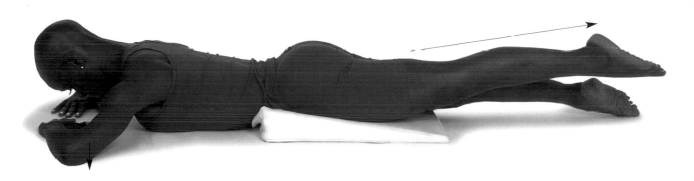

Pincers

Pincers is a variation of the exercise on page 163 and works the adductors and abductors. Remember to maintain the special midpoint lift through the two steps. If you find your lower back aches, stop the exercise and adopt the forward bend (step 4 on page 169). Next time you practise, you will be able to go further.

1 From the start position on page 163, rotate your abductors to turn out from your hips (that is, turn the insides of your thighs and legs towards the floor), point your feet, stretch both legs back toward your feet, and lift from the special midpoint to protect your lower back. Move your feet shoulder-width apart.

2 Now move your heels together until they almost touch. Take a short in-breath, and on a slow out-breath, move your feet a few inches or centimetres apart, then close them. Repeat this movement many times, fast and continuously, beating your heels inward without letting them touch, for eight counts. Rest and repeat three times. Feel the backs of your thighs and buttocks tighten.

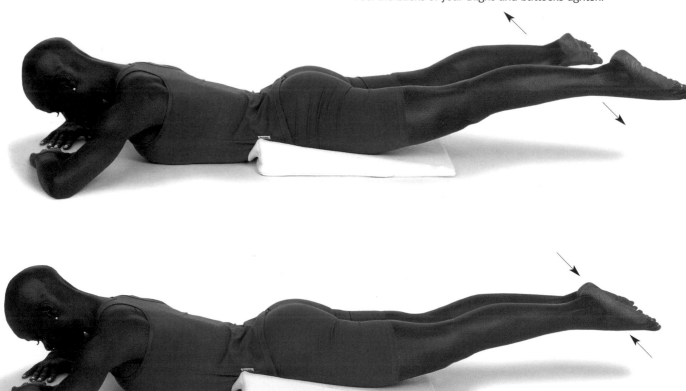

Leg circles

This is an exercise to firm the hamstrings, but it works the buttocks as well. Remember to keep your hips down on the mat through the exercise and to keep them still while you circle and stretch your legs. If your lower back begins to ache, stop exercising, rest for a while in the forward bend position (see pages 169 and 204) and try this exercise again in your next practice.

1 From the start position and on an out-breath, lift your left leg and gently circle it from the hip, four times clockwise and four times anticlockwise. Rest, then circle the right leg.

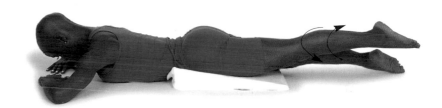

2 Still in the same position, lift your left foot off the mat and stretch it along its length from the sitting bones to the heel.

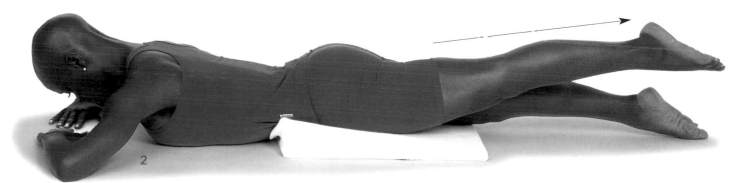

3 Now bend the knee back toward your left thigh, touching your buttocks with your left heel.

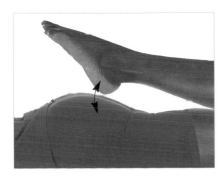

4 Take a short in-breath, and on a slow out-breath, lift your left knee off the mat without arching your lower back. Hold this position for six counts and then stretch out the leg as in step 2. Repeat six times and rest.

5 Repeat steps 1–4, circling and stretching the right leg and lifting the right knee, then rest.

Loosening the hips

Some of the earlier hip exercises were carried out lying on the back. In that position the back is supported and it is easy to keep the hips still. This exercise is more difficult: because you are on all fours, you have to use the transversus abdominis and hamstring muscles to support your lower back while keeping your hips still. In steps 3 and 4, move your bent leg from the hip joint as a unit, keeping the foot strongly pointed and in line with the lower leg. Remember to keep your head and the back of your neck in line with your spine throughout, and to keep your lats and pecs pulled down.

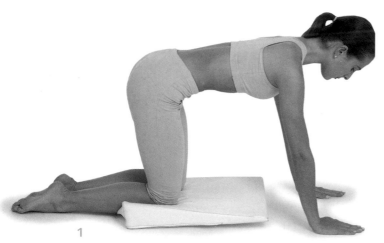

1

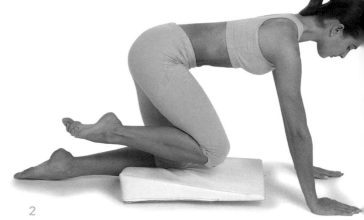

2

1 Kneel on all fours, centering your hips above and slightly behind your knees, and your hands slightly in front of your shoulders. Press your shins and feet down on the mat. If kneeling is painful, rest your knees on a thin cushion, and if you get cramps in your feet, put another cushion or a rolled towel under your ankles, and start again.

2 Apply the special midpoint lift, so your transversus abdominis muscles pull your stomach up towards your lower back. Raise your right knee off the floor without moving the supporting hip and knee, point your right foot hard, and move your knee towards your chest.

3 Circle your right knee out to the side and back, behind you. Rotate from the hip and lift the knee as high as you can so you draw a big circle with it. Keep your left hip directly over your left knee – do not let it swing outwards.

4 Finally, stretch your knee right back, until your trunk and raised thigh form a straight line parallel to the floor and your toes point to the ceiling.

5 Return to the step 1 position and repeat steps 2–4, circling your right leg forwards, out to the side, back, up, and back to the step 2 position in a smooth movement. Remember to rotate from the hip, to lift the knee high, and to keep the supporting knee and hip still. Repeat four times.

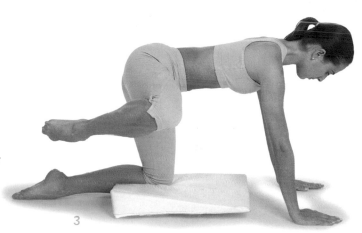

3

Rest and repeat

Return to the step 1 position and rest, then repeat steps 1–4, lifting and circling your left knee five times. Then stretch your leg out, and rest.

Variation

When you are familiar with the exercise and can circle the leg smoothly, repeat it in reverse, circling each leg from the hip: back, out to the side, and forward to the chest.

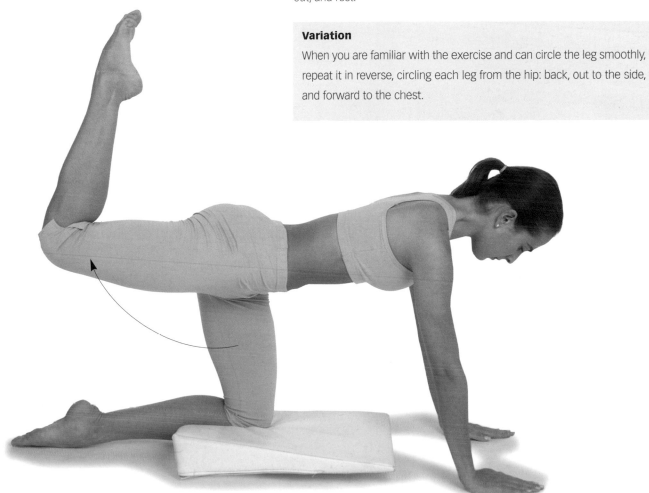

4

Firming the seat

The last three exercises are integrated in this one, which exercises the hamstrings and lower back, as well as firming the buttocks. Keep the supporting knee and hip still, and support your lower back by pulling up from the midpoint using the special midpoint lift. Keep the foot of the raised leg pointing strongly and in line with the lower leg, the lats and pecs pulled down, and the spine, the back of the neck, and the head in line throughout.

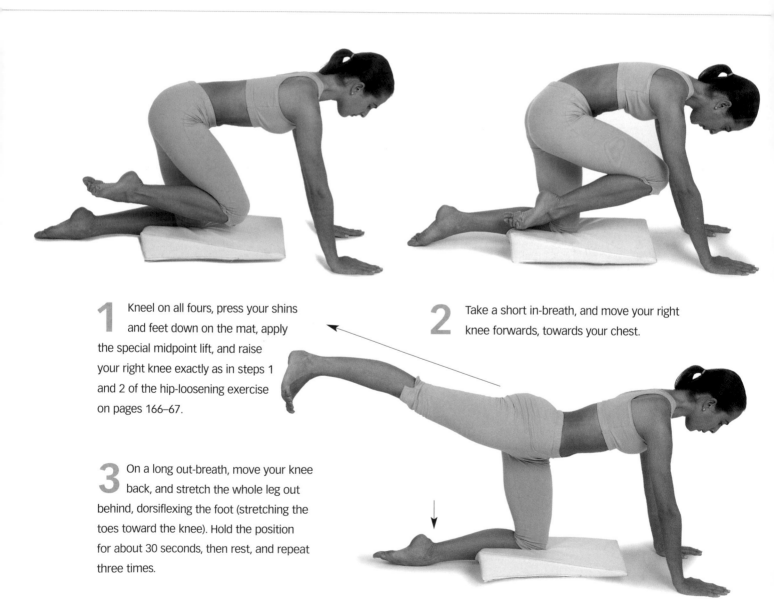

1 Kneel on all fours, press your shins and feet down on the mat, apply the special midpoint lift, and raise your right knee exactly as in steps 1 and 2 of the hip-loosening exercise on pages 166–67.

2 Take a short in-breath, and move your right knee forwards, towards your chest.

3 On a long out-breath, move your knee back, and stretch the whole leg out behind, dorsiflexing the foot (stretching the toes toward the knee). Hold the position for about 30 seconds, then rest, and repeat three times.

4 Repeat steps 2 and 3 three times, then kneel and bend forwards, resting your forehead, forearms and hands on the floor.

Repeat and rest

When you are ready, repeat steps 1–4, this time raising your left knee, moving it forwards to your chest, and stretching your left leg back four times. Then rest as in step 4.

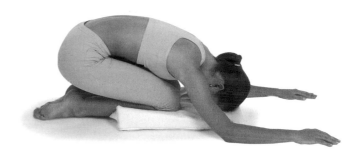

Variation

Repeat steps 1 and 2, then keeping your right knee bent, stretch your right leg out behind you, dorsiflexing the foot, so the sole turns up to the ceiling. Pull up from the midpoint to enable the transversus abdominis muscles to support your lower back. Hold for 30 seconds, then lower your leg so you are kneeling on all fours. Repeat, moving your left knee forwards to your chest then stretching it back, keeping the knee bent. Repeat this variation four more times, then rest as in step 4, and finish.

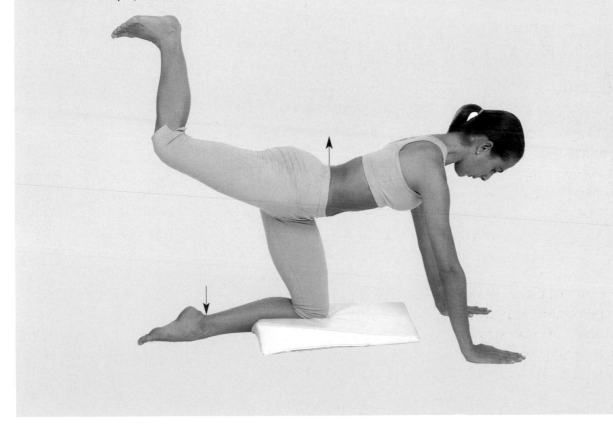

Level 2 Review

Level 2 finishes with the integrating exercise opposite. By now you should be more coordinated and have greater control. Improved coordination comes from integrating the special midpoint lift into every exercise, and better balance indicates that this is becoming second nature. The exercise on these two pages reviews this aspect of Level 2 by comparing a simple hip swivel without midpoint control – as you would have done it at the beginning of Level 1 – with the same movement using the special midpoint lift. For exercises to be effective, you need good balance, and this is achieved by coordinating the body through the midpoint. The more exacting Level 3 exercises require you to lift and hold through long movement sequences.

Integration

Pulling up from the midpoint has the effect of balancing the contribution of all the joints involved in a movement. This is integration – the coordination of messages through the sensors in the joints to the brain – and it gives you the feeling of harmonious movement, as if all parts of the body are working together.

Monitoring posture

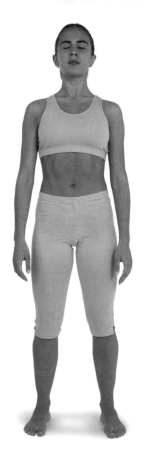

You achieve postural balance by using the joints, but also the special midpoint lift, which enables you to lift your pelvic floor muscles towards the centre of gravity between the hips. This strengthens and supports the hammock formed by the pelvic diaphragm, better enabling it to hold the abdominal organs in their correct position.

1 Stand with your feet apart and parallel, your knees relaxed and your arms by your sides. Your hips, pelvic floor and special midpoint are relaxed.

2 Circle your hips three times to the left without trying to control the movement. As you circle, think about what is happening in your ankle, knee and hip joints. Are their movements smooth and coordinated? Does the spine feel supple, or are you holding it stiffly? How are you holding your head on your neck?

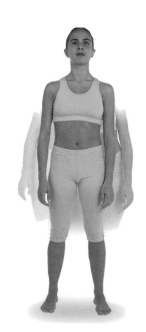

1

2

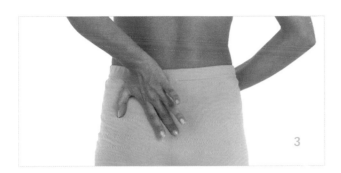

3

3 With your hips still, place your left palm, fingers pointing down, over the joint between your sacrum at the base of your spine, with your middle finger touching the curve of your tailbone. Then cup your lower abdomen with your right hand so that its edge presses against the lower abdominal muscles. If you are left-handed, reverse the positions of the hands.

4 Push both feet with equal pressure against the floor and lift very lightly from the special midpoint, concentrating on the centre of the figure 8 (see page 134), and only just engaging the muscles. Hold, visualizing the transversus abdominis muscles tightening slightly, the tailbone pulling a little farther down and under, changing the angle of the pelvis. Feel your lower back stretch. Your spine should feel connected all the way up, opening at the two top cervical vertebrae, the atlas and axis.

5 Relaxing the special midpoint, repeat step 2, swivelling the hips without controlling the muscles. Then, pushing both feet against the floor, lift the special midpoint lightly and hold the lift while circling the hips again, slowly to the left three times, then slowly to the right three times. Feel the difference between circling while lifting and circling with the midpoint relaxed.

6 Repeat step 5, this time closing your eyes to concentrate more deeply, and compare the two movements. You should notice that circling while lifting the special midpoint gives greater integration of the joints and better control of the muscles from the feet up than when you move without lifting the midpoint. It should make your spine feel more supple, and your head should feel more poised and move more smoothly.

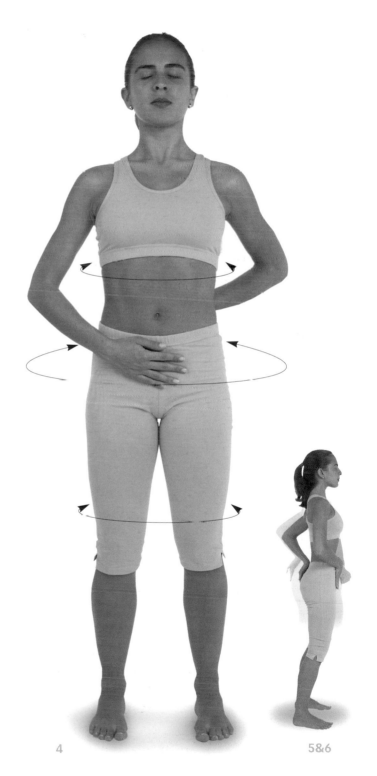

4

5&6

Level 3

Level 3 exercises begin in the seventh week of your rehabilitation and restructuring programme, and if you have completed three exercise sessions a week for the last six weeks you will already notice a difference. Your pelvic floor has been strengthening steadily, bringing a feeling of greater control in and around the abdomen, and improving your posture. Muscle tone has built up, making your body feel stronger and lighter, and the tension around your neck and shoulders has eased, so your upper body feels more relaxed. Your balance is improving, so your movements are becoming more graceful and your body feels better able to counterbalance gravity. This is the time to move to the next stage. Level 3 exercises develop structural fitness.

In essence, to develop fitness is to realize the body's physical potential. In practice, this means that the body assumes its natural shape. At this stage, you must be realistic. The body is never the same for very long. It changes as it matures from youth to adulthood, and during maturity it changes in response to work, parenthood, ageing, posture, injury and lifestyle. The exercise programme in this book will also change it, but how? The body that emerges during Level 3 may not be your body of ten years ago, as you remember it, or the cool image of a model or a celebrity displayed as an ideal in the media.

Your body shape

During Level 3 it may be important to stand back and let your body shape itself. It may not emerge quite as lean as your inner image would have it, but it will not sag, for stronger muscles tighten your profile and make all parts of the body look more shapely. Your legs may not have lengthened to fashion model proportions, but your spine will have stretched, your upper body will have lifted out of your waist, your shoulders will not stoop, and your head and body will sit, stand and walk taller.

As you progress through Level 3 you will inevitably have moments of disappointment. Perhaps your waist is not as shapely as it could be, your inner thighs may still seem flabby. The solution may come from revising Level 1. It may be a surprise to find that these apparently unresponsive parts of the body have, somehow, during the early exercises, been neglected.

We all have blind spots about our body, and the faulty perception extends beyond the reflection in the mirror to the way we move and our approach to exercise. People who feel their upper arms are flabby may hurry through upper arm stretches just because they prefer not to think about their arms. Those with heavy hips and thighs may skimp exercises to stretch, tone and strengthen the lower body because rocking and rotating the pelvis makes them feel ridiculous. Everyone tends to avoid and skimp on the exercises they really need to focus on.

Revisiting Level 1

Overcoming these mental blockages can be hard. One approach is to revisit the first exercises. The most important structural balance exercises are learned in the stages before Level 3, and points may come across that escaped the attention the first time. Moreover, having worked through exercises for six weeks makes the body more receptive, and early exercises may be effective in new ways. If any Level 1 movement still feels difficult, persevere with it. It means that you are really addressing your physical problems, and your body will benefit.

Adjusting to exercise

The structural balance exercises in Level 3 work the body in a range of movements that are achievable for most people, and specially adapted versions and variations are essential for professionals such as dancers and competitors in sports. Although it is hoped that later they will become part of your daily routine, they will be difficult at first, and you will need to help your body adjust. Remember the following points:

Before exercising

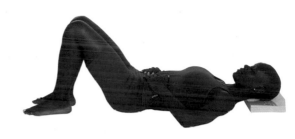

■ If an exercise has caused discomfort or strain, allow yourself a break. Whenever you feel it necessary, roll on your side as illustrated below, then get up and walk around, lifting from the special midpoint for practice during walking. Walk with a comfortable stride, placing your whole foot on the floor, feeling the heel touch down, followed by the metatarsals, and push off from the toes. Your carriage should be easy and natural. Look straight ahead.

Getting up from the floor

■ Sitting up from a lying position can strain the lower back. Always get up from the floor by rolling on one side, then resting your body on your hands as you raise yourself.

Resting position

■ After a particularly strenuous exercise and after a session, always relax. Lie on your back with your knees bent, perhaps over a cushion, and a cushion under your head. Move your feet apart so your knees fall in and may touch, but turn your toes inwards, so you do not stretch the ligaments inside the knees. Breathe in, fold your arms over your chest, and rest for six long, slow out-breaths. Roll to one side to get up, then walk around.

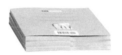

Aids to relaxing

■ Try to end a full exercise session with 15–20 minutes of complete relaxation (see pages 204–05). Placing a foam wedge beneath your head to maintain its correct alignment with the spine, and a triangle to support your knees will relax your body very effectively.

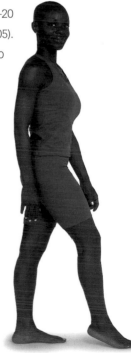

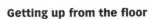

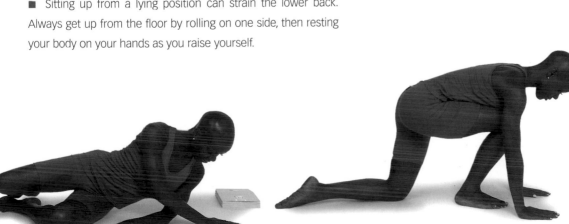

Neck and upper back

These neck exercises strengthen and coordinate the muscles that balance and integrate the movements of the head. Eating, speaking, swallowing, breathing and enjoying a full field of vision when upright or lying down all depend on the balanced functioning of these muscles. They correct the tendency to poke the neck and chin forwards, raising the shoulders, and discourage the habit of hanging the head, burying the chin in the chest, and rounding the shoulders. In time, such postural habits become permanent. Instead, these exercises train you to hold your head high, while keeping your shoulders down and relaxed.

Preparatory exercises

These preparatory exercises are intense, but simple and effective in strengthening the neck muscles. They can also be done at a desk to relieve stiffness caused by prolonged sitting in front of a computer.

Side stretch

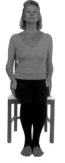

Start position
Sit on an upright chair with your feet together and your hands on your thighs. Pull up from the special midpoint, and press your feet lightly against the floor, heels touching and pressing inwards. Keep your shoulders and lats pulled down.

From the start position, press the fingers of your right hand together and touch the right side of your head, just above the top of your ear, with your palm and fingers. Point the elbow out to the side and sit tall, feeling the upward stretch from the thoracic vertebrae to the atlas and axis. On a slow out-breath, press your head against your hand, and resist its pressure with your palm to a slow count of six, then lower your right hand to your thigh. Rest and repeat four times.

Repeat and rest
Repeat the exercise four times, this time pressing the left side of your head with your left palm and fingers, and resisting the pressure with your head, then relax.

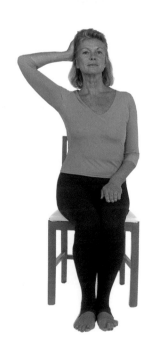

174

Forward stretch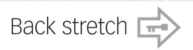

1 From the start position opposite, press the fingers of your right hand together and touch the centre of your forehead with them. Point your right elbow out to the side, keeping the shoulder and lats on your right side down.

2 Stretch your neck up and breathe in. Breathing out to a count of six, press your forehead against your hand and resist its pressure with your fingers, then lower your right hand to your thigh. Rest and repeat the movement four times.

Repeat and rest
Repeat four times, touching your forehead with your left hand.

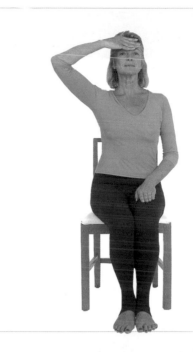

Back stretch

1 From the start position opposite, raise your hands and place the fingertips of both hands together, palms facing, tips of the middle fingers touching.

2 Raise your hands, fingertips touching, over your head and rest them against the back of your neck, the tips of the middle fingers touching in the hollow where the neck meets the head. Open your shoulders and point your elbows outwards in line with your ears. Drop your head forwards and take a short in-breath.

3 On a long out-breath, slowly raise your head, stretch your neck up, and press your head back, meeting and resisting the pressure with your fingers. Stop pressing and look straight ahead, your chin pointing down. Hold this position for a slow count of six, breathing normally.

Rest and repeat
Lower your hands to your thighs, rest briefly, then repeat steps 2 and 3 four times. Feel your spine extend upwards from the middle of your back. Pull your shoulders down and out to the sides. Picture your spine stretching and your head poised and balanced on your neck. Then lower your arms and rest with your hands in your lap.

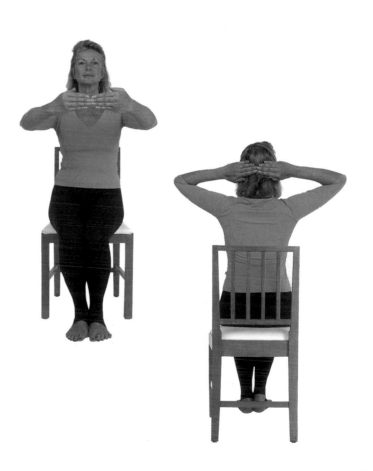

Neck strengtheners

The exercises on these pages strengthen the muscles of the front of the neck, which flex the head, change its angle, and rotate it. By balancing the muscles that make minute adjustments to the position of the head, they encourage good carriage of the head when moving and lying down. They also train you to level your eyes to better assess your surroundings.

Upper back lift

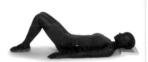

Start position
Lie on your back with your legs together, your knees bent, and your feet flat on the mat. Your arms are by your sides, the forearms and palms of the hands flat on the mat, fingers stretching towards your heels. Rest your head on a book 2.5 centimetres (1) thick to align your neck with your spine. Your shoulder blades should be flat and your shoulders open.

This exercise not only strengthens the neck but it also stretches the upper back. If your breath runs out in steps 2 and 3, take a short in-breath and continue breathing out slowly. If lifting and lowering strain your neck, rest your upper back and head on a thicker cushion so you begin lifting from a higher position.

1 On a slow out-breath, lower your chin to your chest and lift your head off the mat, focusing your eyes on a point between your bent knees. As you do so, touch the xiphoid process (see page 96) with the fingertips of your right hand.

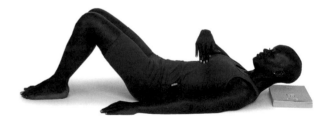

2 Still breathing out, lift your shoulders and upper back off the mat, curling forwards until the tip of your breastbone pushes downwards, acting as the fulcrum or pivotal point of your upper body.

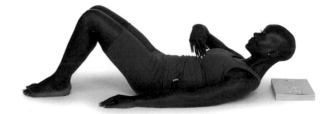

3 Fix your gaze on the point between your knees, and on another slow out-breath, lift your upper body in a controlled movement, and gradually uncurl your back and shoulders to lie back on the mat. Your chin leads down as the back of your head touches the mat. Release your right hand and rest it on the mat.

Repeat and rest
Repeat steps 1–3 four times, release your arm, and rest.

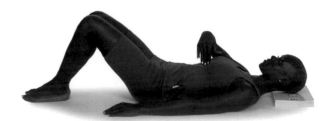

Back-of-the-neck strengthener

Swivelling the head on the axis point while lying on the stomach demonstrates perfectly how we use the muscles at the back of the neck as an extension of the muscles of the spine. By using only the muscles directly involved in an action, you practise perfect economy of movement, which benefits posture and efficiency. Support your stomach on a foam wedge or a pillow in this exercise to prevent any strain to your lower back.

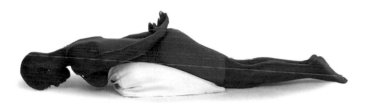

1 Lie on your stomach with your feet stretched back, your forehead touching the mat, and your arms by your sides, then bend your elbows to join your hands behind your back, and interlace your fingers.

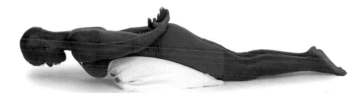

2 Breathe in, and on a slow out-breath, stretch your joined hands and arms out towards your tailbone. Your shoulders lift, aligning with your ears and hips and opening out, your spine stretches out from shoulders to hips, and your hips remain still. Hold for up to 30 seconds.

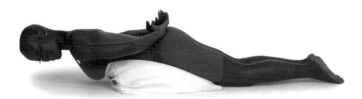

3 Take a short in-breath, and keeping your chin tucked in so your head is in line with your spine and your eyes look down at the mat, turn your head slowly to the left, then back to the centre.

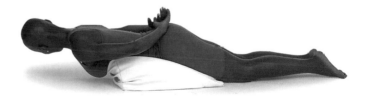

4 Continue the movement, turning your head slowly to the right … and back to the centre…and stop.

Rest and repeat

In a controlled movement, lower your forehead to touch the mat, uncurling your back and following with your shoulders and arms. Rest for a moment, then repeat the exercise six times, and relax.

Lower body

From toning and strengthening the upper torso, Level 3 moves down the body to exercise and shape the waist and abdomen, the lower back, the legs and the feet. After the special analysis of the pelvis in Level 2, this stage focuses on integrating the torso with the lower structures of the body especially. The aim is to develop core strength. Strong muscles in the lower abdomen are essential to maintain a balanced relationship between the pelvis and lower back. This relationship affects all physical activities, from standing to walking and complex sporting activities.

Lower back relief stretch

The lower back tires easily, especially if the transversus abdominis muscles of the lower abdomen are not strong, and in anyone who neglects to exercise. This exercise works and stretches the lumbar spine – usually the part of the back that begins to ache first when you are tired. To do it effectively, take it slowly, concentrating on keeping your spine stretching from the sacrum to the neck. Step 2 demands a lot of effort – to lift your lower back just 5 centimetres (2 inches) off the mat is an achievement and few people can raise it more than 10 centimetres (4 inches). As your tailbone and sacrum rest flat on the floor in step 3, focus on feeling the width of your pelvis from hip to hip.

1 Lie on your back on the mat with your head resting on a book about 2.5 centimetres (1 inch) thick, so that your neck is lengthened and your chin is in a neutral position, inclined towards your chest. Your arms are stretched out by your sides on the mat. Bend your knees and move your feet together.

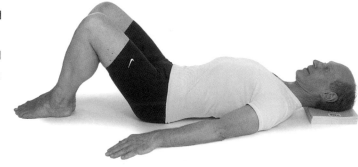

2 Put your hands on your knees and press them down gently towards your body to bring your knees closer to your chest, and lift your feet from the floor. Take a short in-breath, and as you start breathing out, lift the special midpoint so your lower stomach muscles contract. These actions lift your tailbone slightly off the mat, making your lower body curve up.

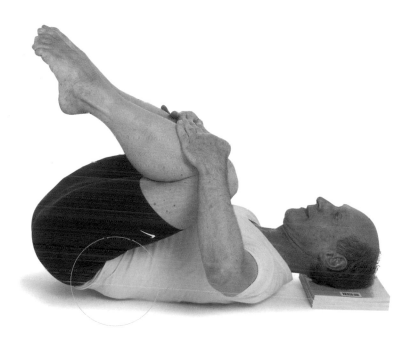

The flexible spine

The large lumbar vertebrae of the lower back are moved by small muscles attached to them on either side. Each pair of vertebrae and each muscle has only a limited range of movement, but they work in unison to arch and straighten the lower back. The 5th lumbar vertebra is fused to the sacrum, which forms the back of the pelvis and does not move. The tailbone consists of four fused bones and moves a little when you lift the pelvic floor and special midpoint.

5 lumbar vertebrae

sacrum

coccyx

3 Lessen the pressure of your hands on your knees, roll your spine slowly back to the floor until your lower back rests on the mat, then straighten your spine and press your shoulder blades against the mat. On a slow out-breath, lift from the special midpoint and stretch along the length of your spine, from neck to tailbone, without arching the middle back.

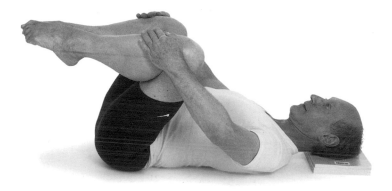

Repeat and rest

Repeat steps 2 and 3 four times, then lie and relax for a while before rolling on to one side and standing up.

Toning the abdominals

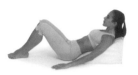

Start position
Sit tall, then bend your knees, draw your heels together, and roll back keeping your head and chest up, until you rest on your lower back with your shoulders open and your arms by your sides. Fall back from the midpoint using the muscles of your lower body. A foam wedge or two cushions placed behind you prevents you falling so far back that you lose control of the midpoint.

The abdominals (often just called the 'abs') – the rectus abdominis and the external and internal obliques – are powerful muscles involved in actions such as bending and rotating the trunk (see page 53). Keeping them taut has a significant aesthetic effect because loss of tone causes the abdomen to bulge, but they also play a key part in core stability. The exercises on these pages improve the tone of your abs and prepare you for the intensified strengthening exercises on pages 188–91. This toning exercise is most effective if you keep your shoulders open and your neck relaxed. Support the weight of your head on your hand without pulling your neck and head forward.

Using a support
In several floor exercises, you need to lift your upper body from the midpoint. Resting against a support, such as a foam wedge 30 centimetres (12 inches) high, enables you to lift and lower from the midpoint and relax the muscles of the upper back and neck. Two fat pillows are an alternative, but a foam wedge (a foam supplier will cut one for you from a block) gives more solid and stable support.

1 From the start position, push both feet with equal pressure against the floor, pressing your heels together and keeping your head and chest up. Lift your right foot and rest the outside of the ankle across your left knee. Raise your left hand and place it behind your head to support its weight, but do not allow your left shoulder to rise to your ear. Instead, keep your lats down and your shoulders open. Your right hand remains stretched out beside your right hip. On a long out-breath, lift from the special midpoint.

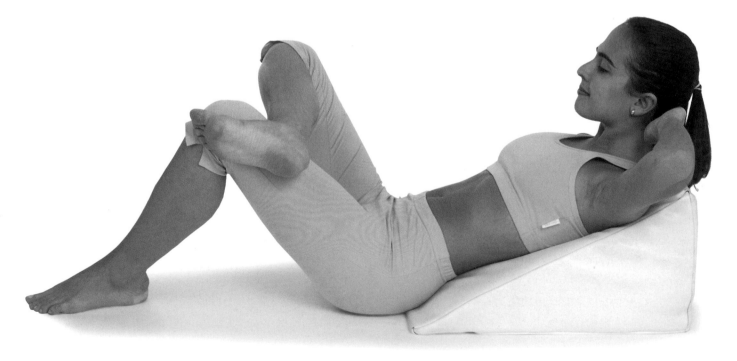

2 Still supporting your head with your hand, and without pulling or straining your neck, raise your upper body from the fulcrum at the xiphoid process of your breastbone, and reach forwards with it towards your right foot. On another long out-breath, focus your gaze directly ahead and lift your left leg until the knee is straightened, pointing the foot.

3 As you straighten your left leg, resist the straightening movement by pressing your right foot against your left knee. Press hard, keeping up the effort for four long out-breaths, then breathe in. Lower your left leg and arm, put your right foot back on the floor, and resume the start position. After a short rest, repeat steps 2 and 3 four times.

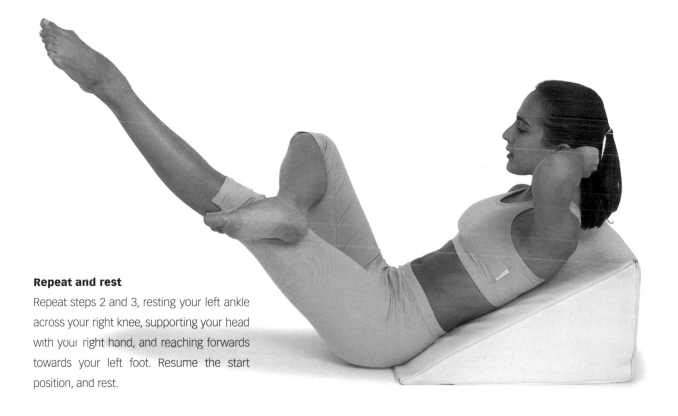

Repeat and rest

Repeat steps 2 and 3, resting your left ankle across your right knee, supporting your head with your right hand, and reaching forwards towards your left foot. Resume the start position, and rest.

Variation

Assume the step 1 position, take a short in-breath, lift from the special midpoint, support your head with your left hand, and turn your torso obliquely towards your right hip. Sustain the effort for three long out-breaths, then lie back and rest. Repeat twice more. Now rest your left foot on your right knee, support your head with your right hand, and turn your torso obliquely towards your left hip. Sustain the effort for three long out-breaths, then sit up and rest. Repeat twice more, then relax.

Foot corkscrew

Visualize a shop dummy when working on the next two exercises. The leg of a dummy may be jointed at the ankle and again at the hip to connect it to the torso. Here, the foot corkscrews from the ankle to work the tendons, muscles and other movable structures that connect ankle and foot to the leg.

Supporting the neck

Several exercises involve lying on the floor. If you lie flat, your head falls back, losing its alignment with the spine, so your chin points up. Support your head and neck on a book or a folded towel about 2.5 centimetres (1 inch) thick, or on a thin foam wedge.

1 Lie in the start position on page 176, and push both feet with equal pressure against the floor, lift from the special midpoint, stretch your spine and flatten your shoulder blades against the floor, opening your shoulders. Lift your right foot and dorsiflex the toes, then, half bending the knee, extend your leg towards the ceiling.

2 Keeping the toes dorsiflexed, dorsiflex the whole foot (pull it upwards) from the ankle, then flex (straighten) it again. Repeat six times, then rest your right foot on the floor beside the left foot.

3 Repeat steps 1 and 2, but lift your left leg and dorsiflex the toes. Now dorsiflex and flex (straighten) your left foot from the ankle six times. Concentrate on dorsiflexing the whole foot, lifting the toes towards the shin, then flexing hard to strengthen the arches. After the sixth repetition, rest your left foot on the mat.

4 Now lift your right foot, dorsiflex the toes, and keeping them dorsiflexed, circle the foot slowly from the ankle, four times anticlockwise and four times clockwise. Rest, then repeat, circling the left foot.

5 Lift your right foot, point the toes hard, and repeat steps 1–4, this time with the toes pointed throughout. Then place both feet on the floor and relax, knees bent, before rolling on to one side, getting up, and walking around.

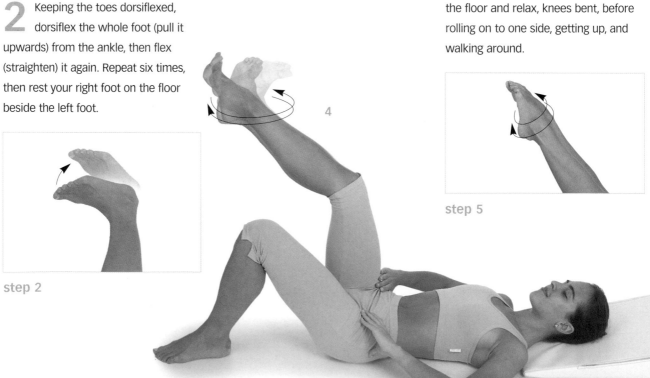

step 2

4

step 5

Single leg corkscrew

In this movement, imagine your whole leg hinged at the hip joint as you circle it inwards, then outwards, involving all the leg muscles. Concentrate on both freeing and controlling the movement of the whole leg, working only the hip joint, keeping your hips still and level, and pressing both hips down on the floor with equal force.

1 From the start position on page 176, push both feet with equal pressure against the floor, lift from the special midpoint, stretch your spine, flatten your shoulder blades against the floor, and open your shoulders, then lift your right foot and, half-bending the knee, extend your leg towards the ceiling. Point the foot hard from the ankle.

2 Breathe in, and on a slow, controlled out-breath circle the entire leg and foot as one unit inwards from the hip, (anticlockwise) then outwards (clockwise), keeping the leg muscles tight. Repeat five or six times, circling inwards then outwards. Rest the leg on the mat.

3 Now repeat steps 1 and 2, this time extending your left leg and circling five or six times, first anticlockwise, then clockwise. Then rest, roll on to one side to get up from the floor, and walk about.

Points to watch

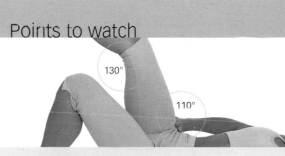

- Raise your leg in step 1 at the point where your thigh forms a 90° to 110° angle to your trunk, and your leg forms a wider angle – about 130° to your thigh. Roughly maintain these angles as you circle your leg – as your leg sweeps round towards you, do not bring it close in, and as it sweeps out, do not bend the knee or let the thigh drop.

Trimming the waist

The long stretch in this exercise works the tensor fasciae latae and the adductors, and the stretch in the variation stretches the quadratus lumborum, the abs, and the gluteals, toning the sides of the body, the abdomen, the lower back, and the thighs. Work at keeping the top leg stretching up in step 3, lifting it level with the uppermost hip and parallel to the floor as shown in step 2.

Supporting the neck

Use a towel to keep your head aligned with your spine in the exercise on these pages and on pages 186–87. Resting your head on your arm raises your head, preventing it from dropping down to the mat, and resting a folded towel on your upper arm and shoulder keeps your shoulders square and your neck and upper back parallel with the floor.

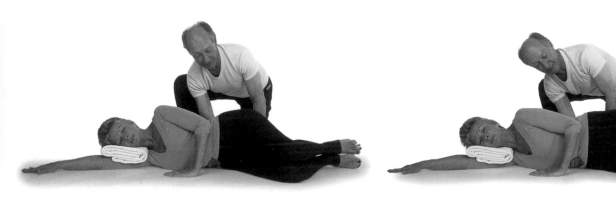

1 Lie on your right side with your right arm stretching out above your head. Place a folded towel on your upper arm and rest your head on it. Your left hand supports your body against the floor, preventing it from falling forwards or back. Your legs are in line with your spine, knees slightly bent.

2 Take a gentle in-breath and apply the special midpoint lift. On a slow out-breath, straighten your left knee, stretch your left leg out in a straight line from the hip, and lift it parallel to the floor. Dorsiflex the foot.

3 On the next out-breath, lift your right foot off the floor and raise it to meet your left foot, then stretch it out from hip to heel, and hold the stretch for two long out-breaths.

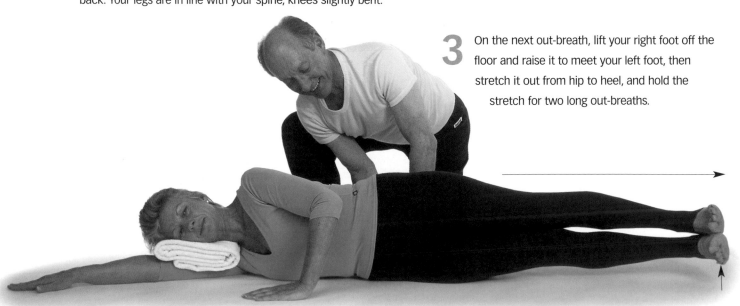

Points to watch

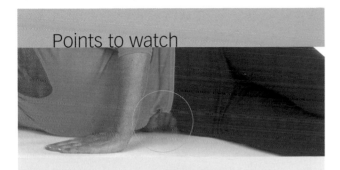

- In steps 1 and 2, keep your waist in its natural position. Do not let it drop down. There should be a gap between the mat and your waist big enough for another person to insert one hand. To maintain that gap, stretch your upper back and neck and keep your shoulders square.

4 Maintaining the stretch, lower both legs to the floor in a controlled movement, keeping the feet dorsiflexed. Relax briefly, then repeat steps 2 and 3 four times, and rest.

5 Turn to lie on your left side and repeat steps 1–3 on a slow, controlled out-breath four times, lifting the right leg and bringing the left leg up to meet it.

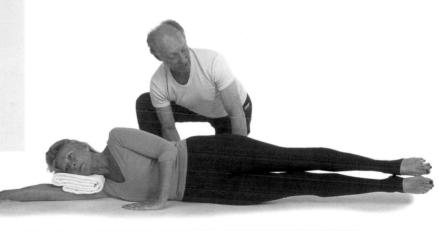

Variation

As you find the exercise becoming easier, raise the level of difficulty by bending your right elbow at the start, and resting your head on your right hand. This makes it easier to let your waist drop down to the floor as you lift your legs, and to let your shoulders slump forwards. Repeat steps 1–5 in this position, and work at keeping your upper body square and your back straight, and keeping the top leg stretching out in line with your spine and parallel to the floor.

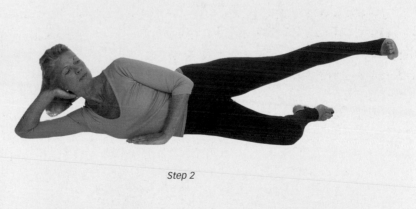

Step 2

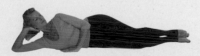

Step 1

Step 3

Scissors

Scissors works the muscles of the waist, the buttocks and the overlapping muscles of the thighs and pelvis. From step 3, extend the backward-moving leg as far back as you can. In this exercise, as in Trimming the waist on pages 184–85, you need to rest your head on a folded towel on your upper arm in order to keep the lower shoulder square and your spine lengthened. Your waist is then lifted high enough off the mat for a friend to be able to insert one hand in the gap.

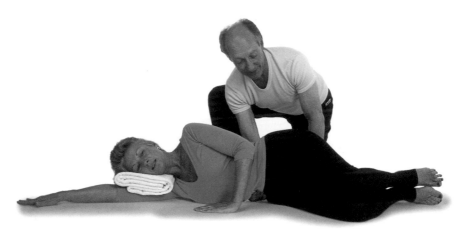

1 Lie on your right side and stretch your right arm out above your head. Place a folded towel on your upper arm to keep the shoulder open, and rest your head on the towel. Place your left hand on the floor in front of you to prevent your trunk from falling forwards or back. Your legs are together, in line with your spine, your knees bent, and your feet dorsiflexed.

2 Keeping your feet dorsiflexed, stretch both legs out in line with your spine. Open your shoulders, lengthen your spine, stretch your legs down towards your heels, and ask a friend to check that there is a gap big enough to insert one hand between the mat and your waist.

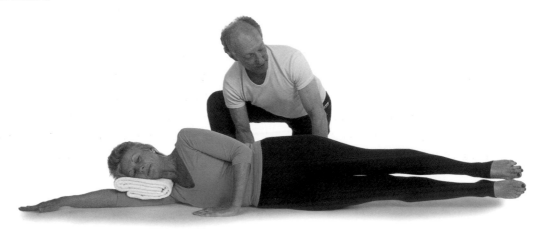

3 Lift your left leg level with your hip. Now practise the scissors movement: first, move the upper leg back from the hip, then forwards from the hip, then back from the hip, then return to the centre; second, raise your right leg, so that both legs are lifted off the mat, and move your right leg forwards from the hip, then back, then return to the centre.

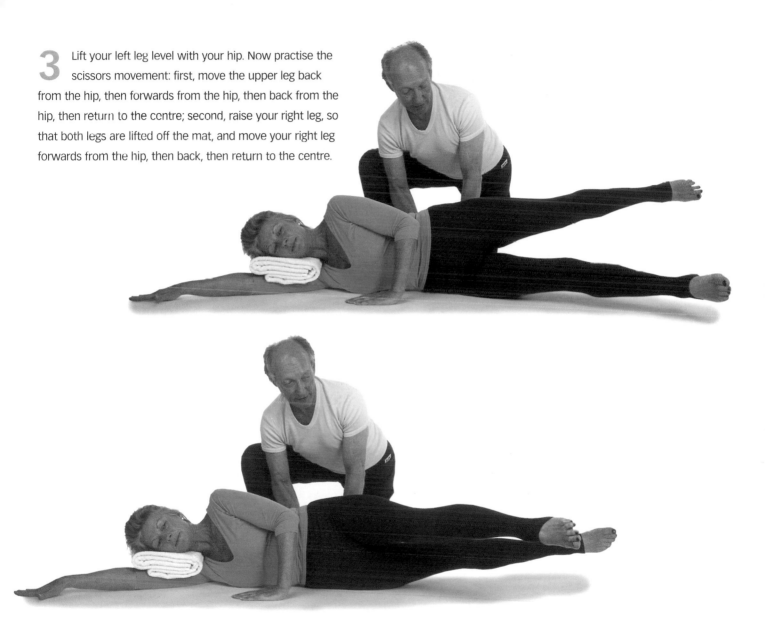

4 Now move both legs in opposition: move your right leg forwards while moving your left leg back, then back while moving the left leg forwards, then forwards again, while moving the left leg back. Bring your legs together again, then stop. Relax, and repeat on a slow out-breath, moving your legs as far forwards and back as you can.

Repeat and rest

Return to step 1 and bend your knees into your stomach. Breathe in, stretch out your legs in line with your spine, and repeat steps 2–4 on the out-breath: scissor three times with controlled, slow leg movements, extending your legs as far as they will go each time, then rest. Repeat three times, then relax.

Strengthening the abdomen

This is a progression from Sitting tall on page 127, since you begin the movement sitting and finish it with your back close to the mat. This exercise stimulates and strengthens the muscles of the lower abdomen, but it is a stage on from Toning the abdominals on pages 180–81. Here you have no support cushion; you have to work at lowering your back all the way down to the mat, using the muscles of your lower body to keep control of the midpoint. When your breath runs out, take a quick in-breath and continue on the next out-breath. As you move back, do not allow your shoulders and chest to collapse inwards, but curve downwards towards the floor, keeping your spine stretching up from the sacrum so that the length of your upper body remains constant.

Wakening the abs

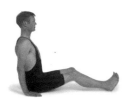

Start position
Sit tall with your knees slightly bent and aligned with your shoulders, your heels together, and your arms by your sides. Lift from the special midpoint. Press your heels together and dorsiflex your feet so your toes point up.

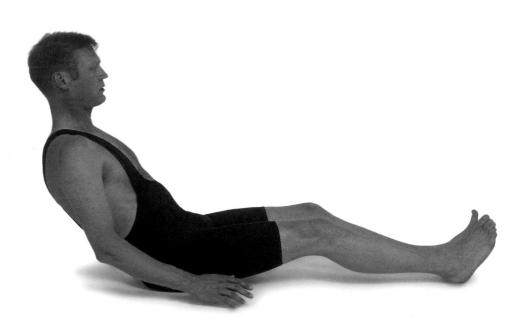

1 On a long out-breath, working from the midpoint, slowly pull the sitting bones under and curve your lower back towards the floor. Simultaneously straighten your legs a little to balance the torso, turning your feet up at a right angle to the floor. As your breath runs out, breathe in quickly and continue steadily breathing out while sinking backwards, one vertebra at a time.

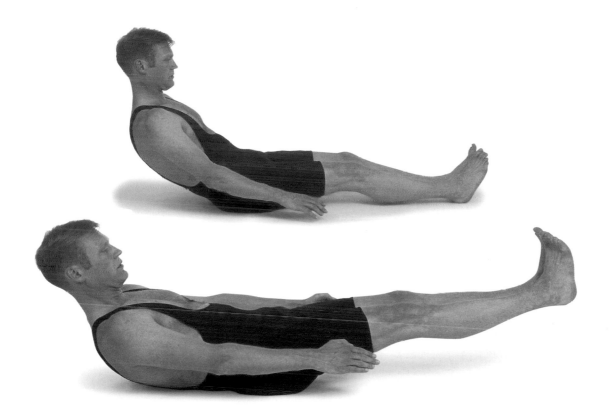

2 Look ahead, towards your toes. As you sink backwards, keep your upper back and chest up, your neck long, and press down from the fulcrum below your breastbone. Let your legs travel forwards slightly, and as they do so, tighten your leg muscles from your buttocks to your heels, and hold.

3 As your breath runs out, tighten the tansversus abdominis and other abdominal muscles, apply the special midpoint lift, and take a short in-breath.

4 On the next out-breath, lower your spine while raising your feet from the floor. Curve your spine only as far back as you can go while feeling totally in control of the movement.

Rest and repeat

When your lumbar spine has reached the lowest point, bend your knees and sit up to take a breather, then repeat steps 1–4 four times.

Points to watch

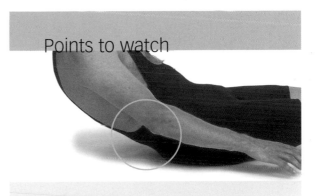

■ When lowering your back in steps 2–4, hold the special midpoint lift while breathing out slowly. Keep your heels together and close to the floor. Your spine should remain curved to prevent strain on the neck. Take it as far back as you can while retaining control over your abdominal muscles. Your lower back stays on the mat through the exercise.

Variation on the Hundred

Joseph Pilates devised the Hundred to work the muscles of the abdomen and the upper back and chest. It is very rigorous and advanced for anyone in their first 12 weeks of practice. This is my version. It flattens the stomach and gives men an impressive six-pack, but few people manage to sustain the lift while counting to 100 without a break. If your muscles start shuddering, or if you feel you are losing control, take two or three breaths, or rest. Do not help yourself with your hands. It is always a good idea to warm up for the Hundred by working through Shaping up, opposite. Keep your knees slightly bent, and your heels and feet pressed together throughout.

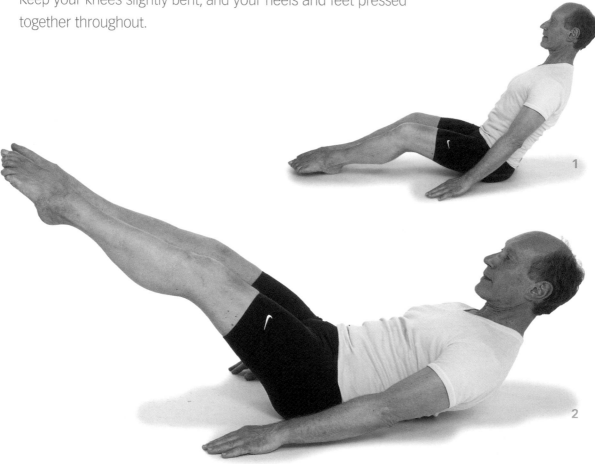

1 From the start position on page 188, press your feet and heels together, breathe in, and on a slow, controlled out-breath, roll back on to your lower back, feeling your lower stomach muscles pull down and tighten. Your lumbar spine folds under, but keep control so you do not fall too far back.

2 Lift your legs about 45 centimetres (18 inches) off the floor without straightening them, and hold, keeping your legs up, while counting to 10 on a slow out-breath, then sit up and rest.

3 Repeat step 2 more than once. Aim at 10 repetitions—so sustaining the posture while counting to 100 on 10 long out-breaths. Beat the timing and rhythm of each count of 10 with your hands on the mat beside your hips.

Finish and rest

When you have completed the last repetition, drop back to the mat, and rest with your knees bent, feet and arms on the floor, breathing evenly through the nose. Then roll on one side to stand up, and walk around, shaking your shoulders and arms.

Points to watch

- While breathing out, do not hold your body static and rigid, but encourage it to curve from the special midpoint to your feet and the top of your head. Move your head from side to side to relieve tension on the neck. Keep your shoulders open and your lats pulled down.

Shaping up

If your abs are not yet strong enough, you may find the Hundred difficult. Work on this exercise first. The farther back you can lean without collapsing, the stronger your abs. When you can lean back at an angle of 45°, stop practising and work on the Hundred again.

1 Sit a little short of a leg-length from a wall and facing it. Sit up and put your hands on the floor by your sides. Lift your right leg, place it against the wall about 30 centimetres (12 inches) up, and push against it for support. Place your left beside it.

2 Put your left hand on your xiphoid process, lower your chin, and curl slowly backwards. Hold for a count of six while pushing your feet against the wall, and grasp your thigh with your right hand. Then raise your trunk to sit upright.

3 Repeat step 2 four–six times, then sit up to rest, and lower your legs.

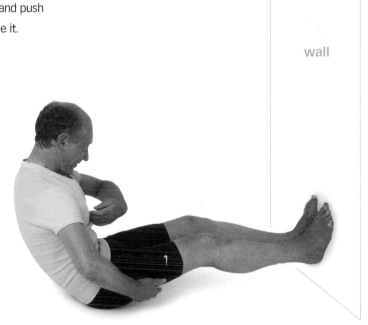

wall

Side hip-lift

Strengthening the upper muscles of the abdomen for better definition around the waistline, and working the adductor muscles of the thighs are the aims of this exercise. You lift each hip and push up on to the elbow, then the feet. You need to build up strength, so begin by doing steps 1–3 on both sides, and attempting step 4 when you feel strong enough. You can also increase the degree of difficulty by raising your left arm over your head in step 2 and the right arm when you repeat the exercise lying on the right side.

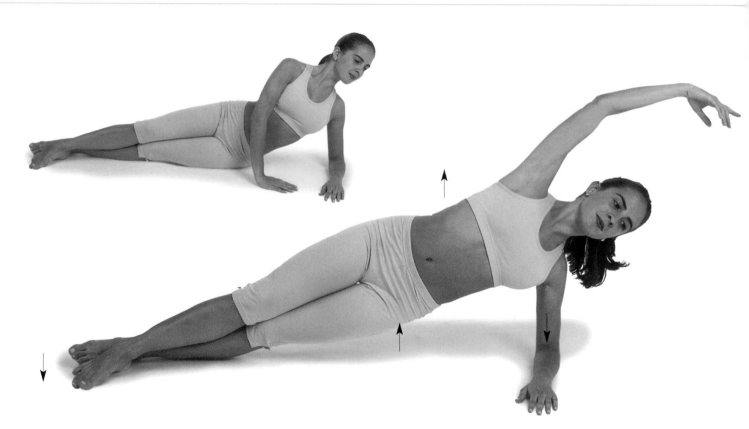

1 Lie on your left side, supporting the weight of your upper body on your left elbow positioned directly beneath your left shoulder and forearm. Your lower body is stretched out on the floor. Rest your right hand on the mat to support your trunk. Cross your right foot in front of your left foot, and press the sole and toes against the floor.

2 Lift your right arm and stretch it up over your head. Breathe in and lift from the special midpoint, then on a slow out-breath, raise your left hip off the floor, stretching your body out to take the weight on the right foot, the right adductor muscles, and the left forearm and elbow. Hold, still breathing out, then lower your hip and relax. Repeat three or four times.

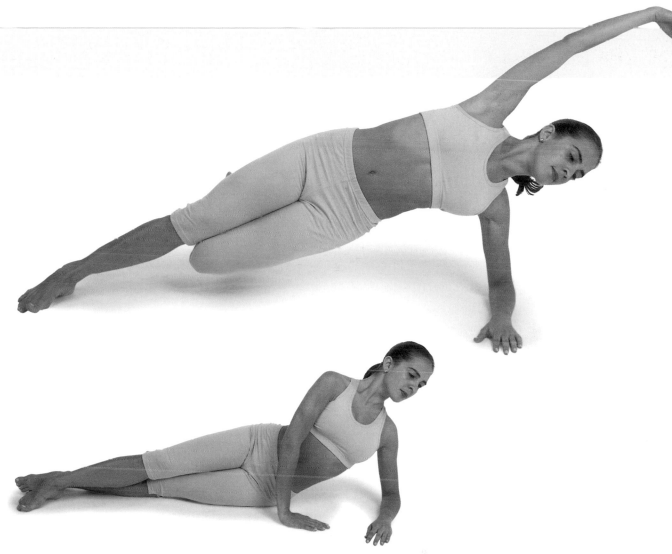

3 Raise your left hip off the floor once more and breathe in. Now bend your left knee, and, if you can, lift it to touch your right knee. Hold, breathing out slowly, then in a controlled movement lower your knee and hip to the floor. Repeat four times, and rest.

Repeat and rest

Turn on your right side and repeat steps 1–3, crossing your left foot in front of your right foot and raising your right hip and knee.

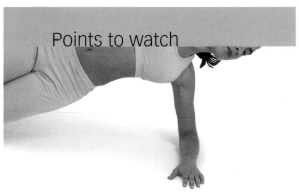

Points to watch

■ In step 3 the supporting elbow should be beneath the shoulder, and your head in line with your spine and slightly inclined, especially if you raise your arm over your head.

Testing coordination

Leg rotation exercises like those on pages 182–83 and here are a good way of improving left-right coordination, something many people find difficult. This is a demanding exercise: you use the special midpoint lift to control the legs from the lower abdomen. Supporting the lower body on a foam wedge (or two fat pillows) makes it easier for a beginner to benefit from doing this exercise before the muscles of the lower body are strengthened. When you feel in control, try it with less support, and work towards doing it lying flat on the mat with no support at all.

Double corkscrew

As well as improving coordination, this complex corkscrew massages the lower back and the lumbosacral plexus, a major junction of nerves travelling from the spine to the lower body. Using the transversus abdominis muscles to control the circling of the legs conditions and strengthens them.

1 Lie on your back, resting your hips and lower spine on a foam wedge, pillows, or cushions, with your knees bent and your arms by your sides. Pull your shoulders down and align your head and neck with your spine. Your chin points to your chest. Now lift your knees and move them in towards your body, raising them level with your special midpoint, then stretch your legs out, keeping your feet above the level of your bent knees. Point your feet.

Rotating the legs

To circle the legs, treat them as if they were a single unit fixed together and hinged from the hips. To get used to this, support them by placing one hand on the outside of each leg close to the knee and using your hands to guide them during the first few circles. Later, place your arms by your sides.

2 Breathe in and press the heels and insides of your feet together. Breathe out slowly, and treating the legs as a single unit, circle them anticlockwise: from the centre of your body, circle them around to the left side, curve them into the waist, circle over to the right side, take them back towards the right hip, and bring them inward to the centre of the body. Repeat this circling twice.

3 Repeat step 2, circling your legs clockwise three times. As you move your legs through the final quadrant of the circle, use the transversus abdominis muscles to stop your lower back from arching off the mat as you reach the end of the out-breath.

Repeat and rest

Rest, then repeat the exercise, circling your legs four times in each direction. Lower your legs slowly to the start position, rest for a moment, then roll on to one side, stand up and walk around.

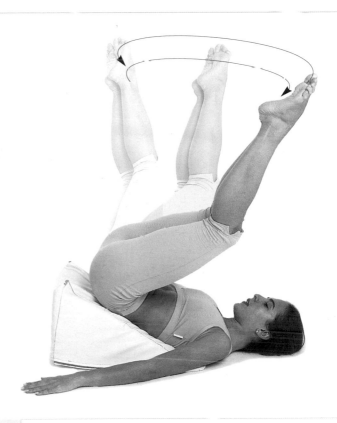

The plexes

Plexes are networks of nerve fibres or of blood or lymph vessels. The body has many, for example, plexes of nerves and blood vessels serve the digestive system. The best known is the solar plexus, a nerve network in the centre of the body just beneath the rib cage. It is one of several major junctions of nerve fibers lying on the midline of the body. The cervical, brachial and lumbar plexes feature in the double corkscrew exercise on these pages.

All body systems are interlinked, so damage to one system reverberates through the body. For example, if the nerves of the lower back are irritated, the internal organs may be affected; a tight psoas may result in constipation. This is why it is essential to learn about how your body functions as you work through the exercises (see pages 24–57). Exercise improves health because it provides an influential link between the nervous and other body systems.

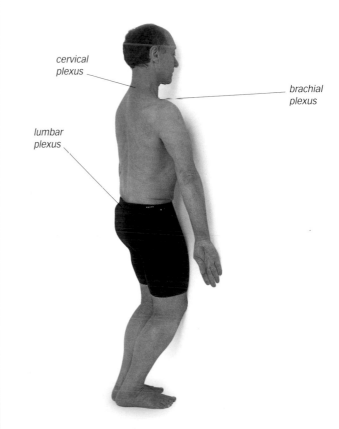

cervical plexus

brachial plexus

lumbar plexus

Lower back bridge

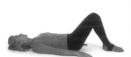

Start position
Lie on your back with your legs together, your knees bent, and your feet flat on the mat. Your arms are by your sides, the forearms and palms of the hands flat on the mat, fingers stretching towards your heels. Your head rests flat on the floor, your neck in line with your spine. Your shoulder blades should be flat and your shoulders open.

The bridge increases the flexibility of the lower back and coordinates the overlapping muscles of the pelvis and legs. If you find it difficult at first, keep trying. When it becomes easier, work the hamstrings and lower back harder by moving the feet farther forwards, away from the buttocks. You should not rest your head on a book or a pillow for this exercise because it would impede the neck stretch, which happens when the pelvis is lifted.

1 From the start position, push both feet with equal pressure against the floor. Apply the special midpoint lift and stretch your spine up. Take a short in-breath, press your heels together, and on a slow out-breath, lift from the sitting bones to raise your lower spine off the mat.

2 Take a short in-breath, and keeping your chin tucked well in and your feet and heels pressing together, press your arms and hands down hard and lift from the midpoint to raise your spine off the mat to form the bridge. Hold, breathing out to a slow count of six, feeling your hamstrings and gluteals contract.

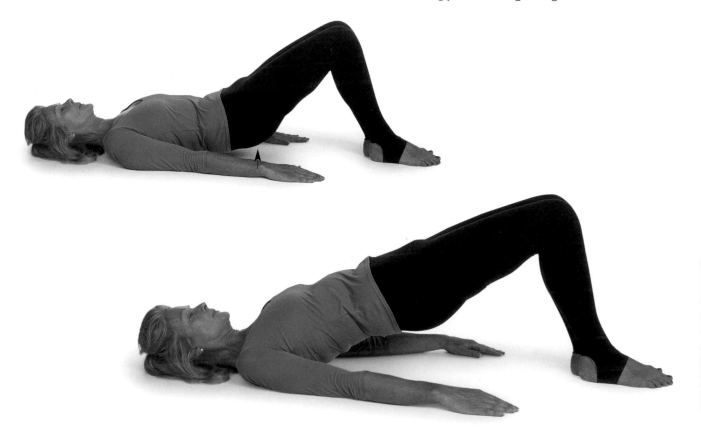

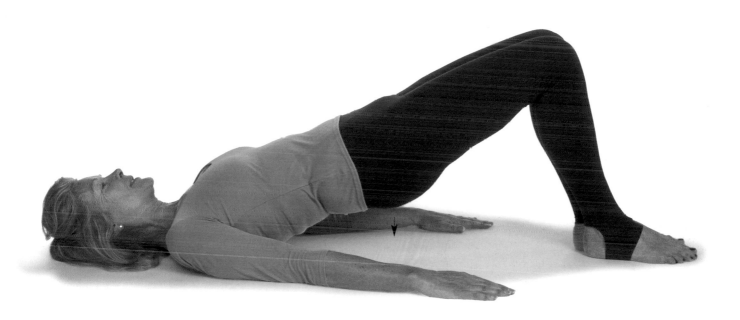

3 Still holding the bridge position, take a short in-breath and contract the transversus abdominis, then breathing out steadily, roll back down to the floor, one vertebra at a time, starting in the upper back and working towards the tailbone.

Repeat and rest

Repeat steps 1–3 four times, lifting the spine slowly on an out-breath, holding while breathing out to a count of six, then taking a short in-breath and lowering slowly, vertebra by vertebra, on the out-breath. Then rest and relax.

Forming the bridge

Never push up on to the neck because this can strain and injure the spine. Lift your spine into a bridge in one movement, pushing up from the sitting bones, not from the lower back, so that one end of the bridge rests on the heels pressing together, and the other on the shoulders. When your spine is raised, your knees, hips, and back are aligned towards the shoulders. Your head and neck should also be in line with your spine, and your head, neck, and shoulders lie flat on the floor throughout.

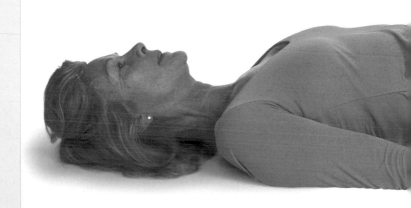

Floating legs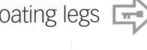

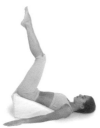

Start position

Lie on your back, resting your hips and lower spine on a foam wedge, pillows, or cushions, with your knees bent and your arms by your sides. Pull your shoulders down and align your head and neck with your spine. Your chin points to your chest. Now lift your knees and move them in towards your body, raising them level with your special midpoint, then stretch your legs out, keeping your feet above the level of your bent knees. Point your toes.

The Double corkscrew on pages 194–95 is an essential preparation for this exercise, in which you lift the pelvis off the floor and balance on the upper torso. It works the lower abdominal muscles and the pelvic area hard. Start by using a foam wedge or two fat pillows to support your hips and lower back, and when you feel more in control, reduce the support until you can do the exercise lying flat on the mat. When you lift your lower spine, try to raise your hips and legs close to the perpendicular without arching your back. This will be easier if you keep your arms by your sides, but work towards doing it with your arms extended over your head. Remember not to lift your chin, but to keep it down and to extend and relax your neck.

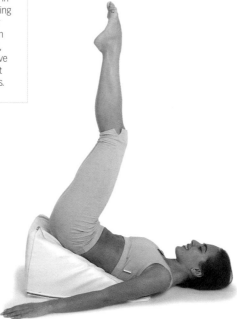

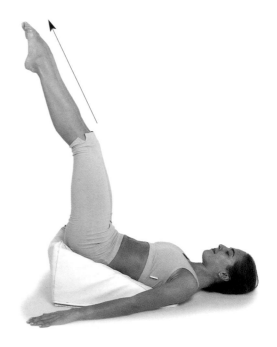

1 Keeping your legs together and your knees slightly bent, stretch both legs up as high as you can, so they almost form a right angle to your torso. Inhale briefly, apply the special midpoint lift, press your heels and the insides of your feet together, and on a slow out-breath, contract your lower stomach muscles and lift your hips off the cushion, supporting your lower body on your arms and on the upper part of your back.

2 Breathe in, and keeping your toes pointing up and your pelvis lifted, reach farther up and away with your feet. Try to hold, breathing out, for 30 seconds, then relax.

Repeat and rest

Repeat steps 1 and 2 six times. To finish, bend your knees to lower your legs to the floor, then roll over on one side, stand up, and walk around before moving on to the next exercise.

Variation 1

When you feel you can lift and hold easily, repeat the exercise, increasing the difficulty: after you lift your lower back in step 1, breathe in and to a slow count of six, hold your legs slightly off the perpendicular at an obtuse angle to the body.

Variation 2

When you can carry out the exercise lying flat on the mat, without supporting your back, try this advanced version. Instead of placing your hands on the floor beside you, raise them above your head and ask a friend to place one hand behind your heels and press hard against them to stop yourself falling backwards.

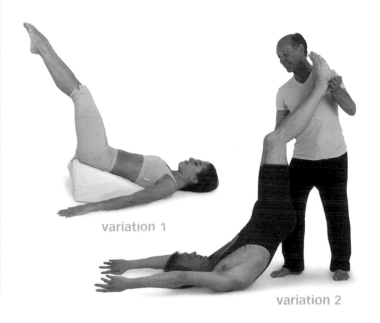

variation 1

variation 2

Low rainbow bridge

Attempt this advanced exercise when you have mastered all the Level 3 exercises up to this point. Low rainbow bridge is the most difficult and complete exercise for integrating and strengthening the muscles of the lower back and buttocks. It works the lower back hardest of all, and it exercises the multifidus. Start with four repetitions, and when you begin to find the exercise easier, proceed to eight.

1 Lie on your back with your arms over your head. Stretch out your body, move your heels together and align them with your hips, and dorsiflex your feet so your toes point upwards.

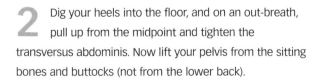

2 Dig your heels into the floor, and on an out-breath, pull up from the midpoint and tighten the transversus abdominis. Now lift your pelvis from the sitting bones and buttocks (not from the lower back).

3 Relax briefly, then repeat step 2 and hold the lift for a count of six, and relax. Repeat four times, then raise your knees to your chest to rest your lower back. Roll on to your side, stand up, and walk around.

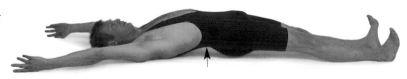

Points to watch

- Keep your legs stretching out and do not draw your heels in towards your body as you stretch.
- You may be able to lift your seat just clear of the floor at first, but work towards clearing a 10-centimetre (4-inch) gap.

Knee-bend rebound and stretch

This exercise is a modest introduction to reactive power and speed against the floor. Its aim is to improve the condition of the ligaments of the knees, ankles and hip joints. It mimics the athlete's rebound from both feet over hurdles and obstacles of various heights and widths, and it contributes to a speedy takeoff for explosive running, sprinting, or jumping. It is an advanced exercise, and the knee bends on page 113 are an essential preliminary to it, since they strengthen the complex muscle structure involved. Exercise against a wall to keep control while timing the rebounds and stretches.

Warning

Rebounds are not for anyone who is overweight or who has had a hip replacement. If you have knee problems or have recently had surgery on the knee, you should attempt rebounds only after thorough physiotherapy for the integration and recovery of the limb. If you are in doubt, check with a physician before trying it.

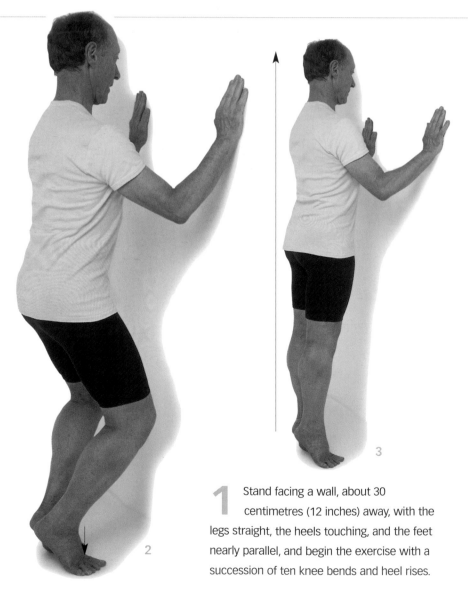

Points to watch

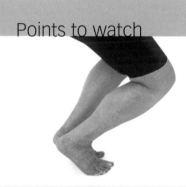

■ Your heels do not bounce but stay about 5 centimetres (2 inches) off the floor and press inwards so the body does not collapse. Use your hamstrings and adductors to move your knees and hips, and bounce up from the ball of the foot. Go gently, and stop if you feel any strain on your knees.

1 Stand facing a wall, about 30 centimetres (12 inches) away, with the legs straight, the heels touching, and the feet nearly parallel, and begin the exercise with a succession of ten knee bends and heel rises.

2 On the next knee bend, press your heels together and bend your knees more deeply until your heels lift off the floor.

3 Now use the rebound to rise into a calf stretch.

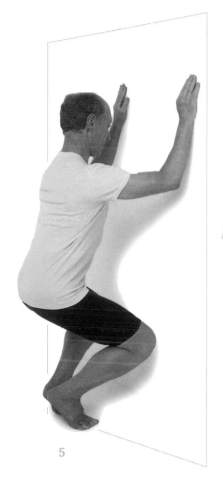
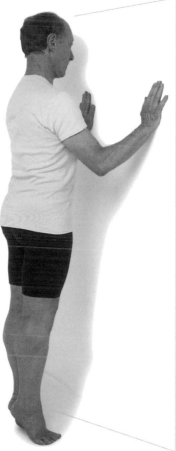

5

4 Repeat step 2 four times, rebounding each time as if on an upbeat. Do it fast, keeping your heels quite still and rebounding up from the balls of the feet, so that your knees and hips move, not your feet and ankles.

5 Repeat the exercise every two days, gradually bending more deeply, and adding one extra rebound each session, until you complete a sequence of ten.

6 Finish with a few calf and hamstring stretches from pages 114, 117, and 120–21. Rebounds tend to shorten the hamstrings and calf muscles, and stretching is needed to lengthen them.

Plyometrics

The rebound is the basis of the reactive kick-start. This sprinting technique was first introduced into athletics training for Valeri Borzov, the 20-year-old Soviet 100-meters champion at the 1972 Munich Olympics. Borzov became the first to run the distance in 10 seconds. The training technique he used, called plyometrics, enabled him to get off to the fastest possible start and accelerate to the maximum sprinting speed in the fastest possible time. Plyometrics uses the stretch reflex (see page 32) to develop the rebound qualities of the feet and legs through exercises. These involve jumping off a surface at one height, rebounding directly onto a higher surface, and again directly onto a much lower surface, and so on, never pausing for rest or recovery.

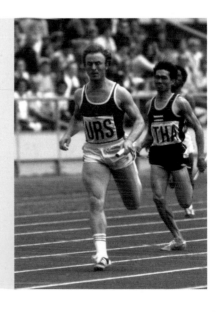

Valeri Borzov, Soviet sprinter, competing in the 1976 Olympic Games in Montreal.

Bear walk

Several exercises on earlier pages focus on lengthening the hamstrings and maintaining their flexibility. The thigh stretches against the wall and from a chair (see pages 118–21) provide a necessary preparation for progressing to the more advanced variation below. This gives the ultimate hamstring stretch, since it works at stretching the heels right down to the floor.

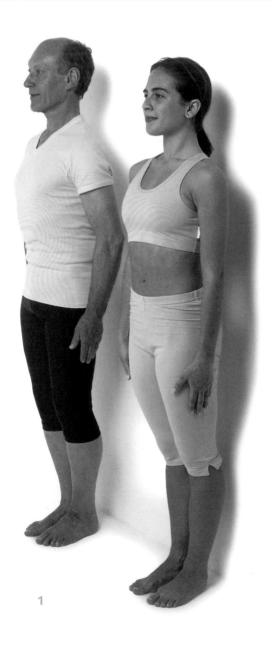

1

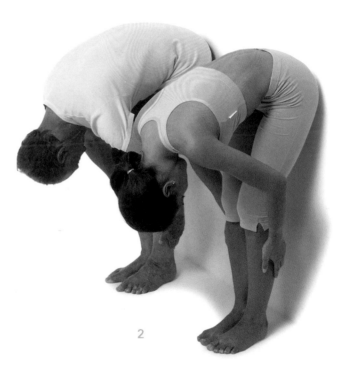

2

1 Stand leaning with your back against the wall, your feet 12–25 centimetres (5–10 inches) away, your legs straight, and your hands by your sides. Press your tailbone and spine against the wall.

2 Tuck in your chin, hang your head heavily, and roll down from your neck, directing your gaze down to your navel and feet. Slide your hands down the sides and backs of your legs as you curl down, continuing as far as your hamstrings will allow, then bend your knees a little to touch the floor with your hands.

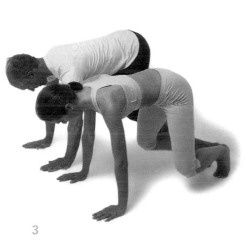

3

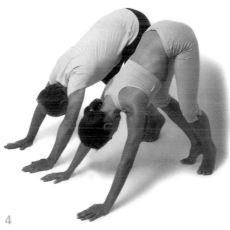

4

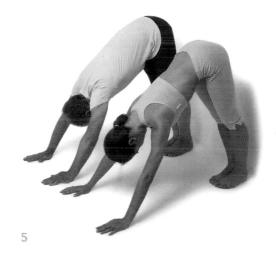

5

3 Without moving your feet, transfer your weight to your hands and move your tail and body away from the wall. Now walk forwards with your hands into the bear stance, bending your knees and pressing your heels together as they lift, until your back is parallel to the floor.

4 Tuck your head down and feel the bear stretch between your shoulders, then straighten your knees as much as you can, ideally until your back is angled down towards the floor.

5 Keeping your legs as straight as you can, walk back to the wall with your hands until your tail and your spine press against it once more, then unroll your spine until you stand upright again. Rest your hands by your sides.

Repeat and rest

Repeat steps 1–5 every day for six weeks, trying each time to lower your heels a little closer to the floor in the bear stance, and to hold the stretch in step 4 a little longer each time, until you can hold it for up to 3 minutes.

Variation

When your heels can touch the floor comfortably, move your feet closer to the wall before standing upright. As your hamstrings loosen, move your feet gradually closer to the wall, keeping your knees straight in the roll down and the unrolling.

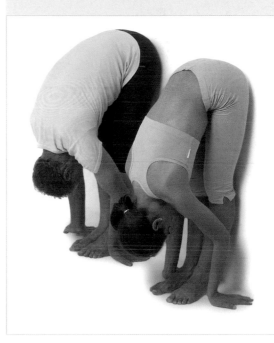

Using the wall

Use the wall to stabilize yourself while rolling down into the bear stance in step 2, trying to keep your nose as close as possible to your body. When you have rolled down as far as you can, put your tail against the wall and roll back up, using your transversus abdominis muscles and the arches of your feet to keep control and balance. When you can do this exercise with your heels about 15 centimetres (6 inches) away from the wall, move your heels closer to it (see Variation), aiming at having them only about 8 centimetres (3 inches) away.

Ending with relaxation

The exercise session began on page 84 with massage, and it ends here, with a short relaxation session. Just as massage prepares the body for exercise by easing away tightness and rigidity in the muscles, relaxation gives it time to recover, allowing the heartbeat to slow to its normal working level and stretched muscles to rest and shorten. Body and mind are inseparable, and complete relaxation after exercise helps the learning process, enabling the mind to review new movement experiences and to sift and store them for future use. And while exercise provides a brief respite from everyday problems, giving them new perspectives, relaxation helps this process by clearing and refreshing the mind, making it easier to adjust from the exercise environment back to everyday life.

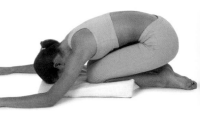

Rest lying on your back with your knees bent and your head supported on a pillow or a folded towel (right). You might also rest your feet on a cushion (far right). Alternatively, relax into a forward bend (below) if you have been practising exercises that work the lower back hard.

It is easy to devise a personal relaxation programme using any one of many thoughtful and penetrating relaxation systems, such as bio-energetics, autogenics, and visualization. This short sequence is perennially popular. After you finish exercising, just lie on your back on the mat with a pillow or a folded towel beneath your head, place your arms by your sides, and close your eyes. Take 15 to 20 minutes to work slowly through this relaxation exercise, repeating each step three times.

I take a gentle in-breath, I suspend my breath…I count one…two…three…four…five…six … feeling the stillness of my body… and I breathe out, letting go gently and completely.

I take a gentle in-breath, I suspend my breath…I squeeze the muscles of my arms and hands into a hard fist …I feel how hard I squeeze …and I breathe out…I allow the muscles of my arms and hands to unfold gently and completely.

I take a gentle in-breath, I suspend my breath….I squeeze the muscles of my toes and feet into a hard arch…I feel how hard I squeeze…I breathe out…I allow the muscles of my toes and feet to unfold gently and completely.

I take a gentle in-breath, I suspend my breath…I squeeze my thighs and my buttocks hard together…I feel how hard I squeeze…and I breathe out…I allow the muscles of my thighs and buttocks to unfold gently and completely.

I take a gentle in-breath, I suspend my breath …. I squeeze the muscles of my face and neck, my eyes and mouth together… I feel how hard I squeeze…and I breathe out…I allow the muscles of my face, neck, eyes, and mouth to unfold gently and completely.

I take a gentle in-breath, I suspend my breath…I squeeze the muscles of my buttocks, pelvis, stomach, and chest hard

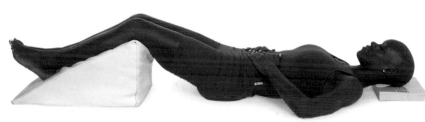

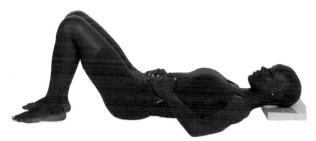

together…I feel how hard I squeeze…and I breathe out… I allow the muscles of my buttocks, pelvis, stomach and chest to unfold gently and completely.

I take a gentle in-breath, I suspend my breath…I squeeze together, strong and hard, all the muscles of my body in one go…my fists…my arms…my feet…my legs and thighs…my buttocks and pelvis…my face and neck…I feel how hard I squeeze. and I breathe out …I allow my whole body to unfold gently and completely.

I breathe gently in and out…in and out. I review my whole body and see how relaxed I am. I confirm that my legs and feet are relaxed…my thighs, pelvis and buttocks…my stomach and

chest…my face and neck muscles…my shoulders.

I imagine I lie in my favourite spot by the sea…I feel my body sink into the warm sand, and I hear the distant sounds of the waves…the gentle sun touches my skin, the soft breeze from over the water…I hear the sounds of birds…I feel my whole body relaxed and refreshed.

If it is night, I can float off to sleep.

But now, I squeeze my fists and stretch out my whole body, from above my head to my toes. I open my eyes and come back to the room refreshed and recovered. I walk around and gently go about my business before I reshoulder` the pressures of the day.

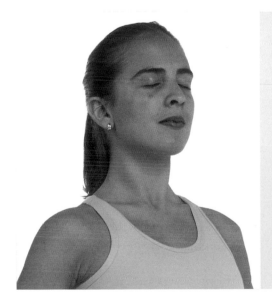

Banishing stress

Mental and physical tensions are entwined in the condition called stress, and bio-energetics, autogenics and other systems use the interaction of mind and body to transport both to a tranquil environment. It is useful to be able to switch off and refresh body and mind at any time, especially when you need to fall asleep peacefully. For serious stress problems causing tension, anxiety, sleeplessness and illness, Autogenic Training is a relaxation therapy based on simple mental exercises that enable you to address the causes of stress quickly, in order to regain power and control. Bio-energetics explores the patterns of energy flow through the body and works on their physical and mental effects.

part 6
specializations

Dreas understands the need of actors
to embody, the need of dancers to perpetually
reach beyond physical limitation.

SALLY POTTER, WRITER, ACTOR, FILM DIRECTOR

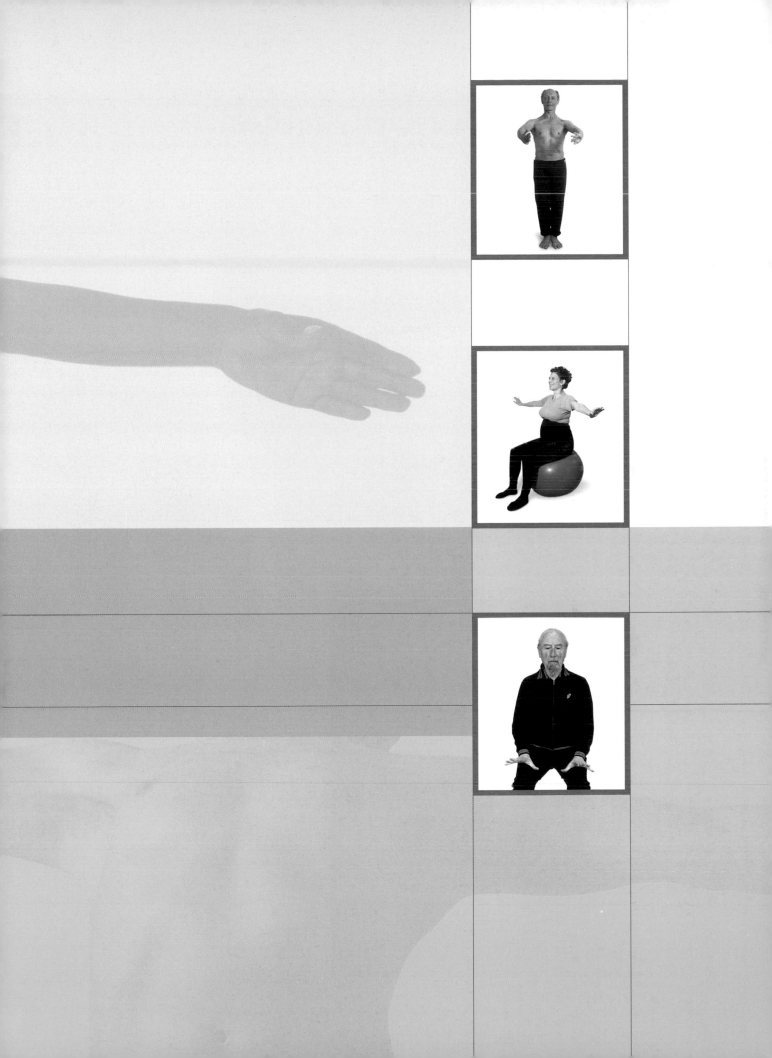

Special adaptations

Pilates is a generalized exercise system that can benefit almost everyone, and seems infinitely adaptable to people's different needs and requirements. It can improve the fitness of men and women in every age group from the late teens into old age. Properly supervised, it can be beneficial during pregnancy and it is a gentle form of exercise for the later decades of life. Pilates can help anyone who plays a sport regularly for recreation or as a profession. And in recent years it has proved its value to the performing arts. I have had the privilege of working with many well-known dancers and actors from the theatre and the cinema, with writers, and with professionals in other creative fields.

Every body's owner needs to keep his or her anatomy and physiology in good working order. This can be hard at first, but the exercises are enjoyable and not stressful, and every dedicated person quickly becomes structurally fit. The exercise programme in Part 5 can benefit anyone old enough to have passed through the adolescent growth spurt. Begun at this early stage and continued through life, it will keep the body supple and mobile into old age.

As two mothers testify on pages 214–15, pilates stretches can be a boon during and immediately after

Among the many musicians who find their work develops one side of the body more than the other are pianists, who use the right hand very heavily and tend to strain the area between the neck and the shoulder on the right side of the body. They need to strengthen and balance the lats and exercise the neck muscles (see pages 103–06 and 175–77).

pregnancy, although to be able to benefit, it is necessary to have started exercising a considerable time before pregnancy begins. There are no exercises especially for pregnant women; instead, the regular programme of the mother-to-be needs to be adapted to the changing body. For this, supervision by a qualified instructor is necessary.

Isabel Fonseca compared the structural fitness exercises she practised during her most recent pregnancy (see page 215) with the exercises she was taught during her first one. She found that the Kegel exercises commonly taught in antenatal clinics—for example, the pelvic tilts, and the often perfunctory leg lifts taught on postnatal wards—tend to be dreary, if not baffling, and contribute little to the general sense of well-being. By contrast, structural fitness exercises, while focusing on this or that body part, also take care of the whole person. 'I always feel wonderful after a pilates session', she remarked, 'energetic, limber, and peaceful, but especially so during pregnancy when mental fitness is as important as the physical, but often more elusive'.

Pilates is one of very few Western exercise systems that people in the later decades of life find attractive and suited to their needs. One of my former clients began in his seventies and continued until his death in his mid-nineties. Pages 216–17 show the range of exercises he found helpful. Older people really need to exercise under professional supervision to plan a programme suited to their personal requirements, and to adapt it as they change. Certain exercises should not be attempted by anyone with a hip replacement, but essentially, everyone,

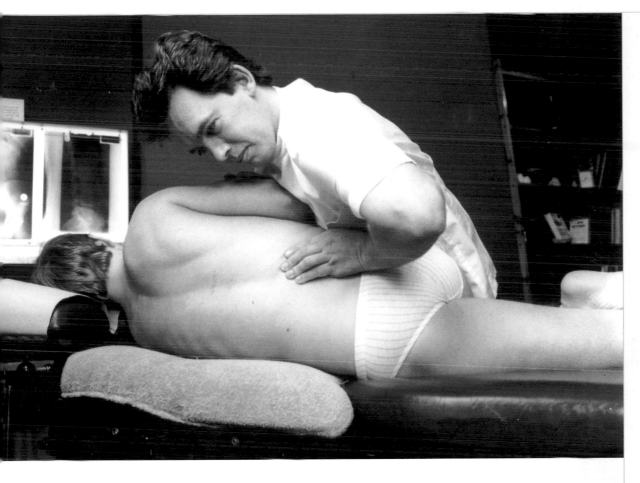

Osteopaths and chiropractors, whose work involves constantly bending forward and pressing down, need to work on opening the chest.

of whatever age, should follow a programme to loosen, stretch, tone, strengthen and balance the body.

I am often approached by dancers requiring help with fine-tuning their body to improve its performance, while actors often need help with moulding their body into a particular role (see pages 210–11). However bizarre the role, the adaptation can usually be achieved, given time. Being called upon to work out ways of helping professionals in these and other, broadly differing fields

with a wide range of body-conditioning problems has been invaluable in helping me develop my exercises.

The exercises in Part 5 are an essential warmup for sports professionals, and effective for recuperation after sports injuries. They help prevent strains and minor disorders caused by sports such as tennis, in which one hand does most of the work. A qualified supervisor can assess the needs of sports players in all fields and adapt exercises to their needs.

A great teacher is one who teaches by their presence as much as by their words. In a lifetime they are very rare and Dreas is one of the finest. VIVIANA DURANTE, PRINCIPAL BALLERINA

Structural fitness for actors

A perfect body is not a prerogative for everyone, however talented they may be, so actors need to work at body-conditioning as much as everyone else. General exercise will often answer their personal and professional needs, especially when they are playing a character whose physical attributes are similar to their own. Sometimes, however, they take on roles that require them to change their body in unusual ways. Structural fitness exercises have enabled many actors to mould their body into unfamiliar forms, to adopt an unaccustomed gait and posture, and even to communicate in a different body language.

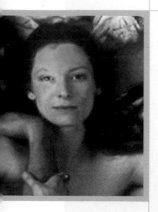

Tilda Swinton changed from woman to boy in the film Orlando, *and her self-expression had to change with it. Structural fitness training at the Body Conditioning Studio helped her adapt her stance, gestures, and gait for the scenes in which she played a boy.*

Actors often have very specific requests, so for them body-conditioning may need to involve more than merely keeping fit. I am frequently consulted by actors wanting help in shaping their body to fit a character whose natural physique does not correspond with their own. For example, because the body has changed considerably over historical time, actors cast as characters of the past may need to adjust their body proportions in order to fit into the role. It is not always as easy as dressing to look the part. For instance, the muscular arms of a female actress who regularly works out scarcely look as if they belong inside the sleeves of a day dress belonging to an indolent, 19th-century lady of fashion.

Film actors sometimes need to make more radical changes. The French actor Christopher Lambert prepared for the role of Tarzan, for Hugh Hudson's film *Greystoke: the Legend of Tarzan, Lord of the Apes* at my studio. The brief was to change his body from that of a French intellectual educated at the Paris Conservatoire, to that of an individual whose life had been spent learning to swing from trees and live as an animal.

Neither men nor women look the part in period costume if they are too built up. Rather than develop muscular arms and shoulders for her boy part in Orlando, *Tilda Swinton concentrated on practising and perfecting male body language.*

Whatever the request, the first priority is always to balance the body structurally. In the past I have followed the pattern of improving posture and the confidence that naturally accompanies the physical changes. Once the body is balanced, other aspects of the prospective acting role are brought into play and its specific requirements addressed. The next step is to work on the body language required for the role. I always find it rewarding when my contribution is seen as valuable to that aspect of a role as well. An actor will often continue developing and conditioning the body long after the role that brought him or her to the studio is over. And many will soon return to work on the adaptation for another, different character.

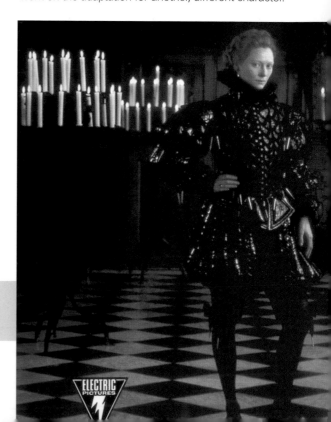

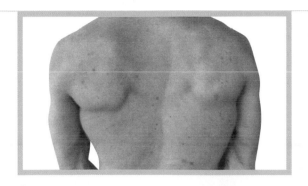
1

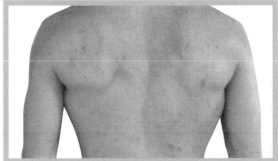
2

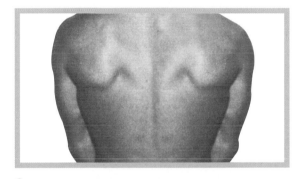
3

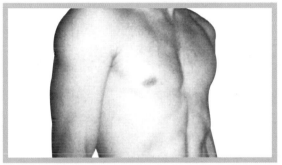
4

Tarzan of the Apes

The French actor Christopher Lambert transforms his body into that of a Tarzan for Hugh Hudson's film *Greystoke: The Legend of Tarzan, Lord of the Apes*. The brief was that he had to be 'long and stretched, with an overall body development that shows how active his life has been...swinging from the trees and living as an animal'. It ruled out pumping iron, which works fast, but its uniform muscle development belies its origins in the metropolitan gym. A curvature of the spine badly affected his posture and raised one shoulder higher than the other. The first priority was to balance the body structurally before putting on muscle, which would have worsened the postural problem or even have resulted in injury. Two intense sessions a day realigned his shoulders, then work began on remodelling the muscles of his limbs and torso to create the look of a lifelong jungle-dweller in just five months.

1 Week 1: *note the high shoulder blade and the curvature at the top of the spine.*
2 Week 6: *the shoulder blade is returning to its natural position and the upper spine is straightening.*
3 Week 12: *the upper spine is straight and the balance of the shoulder blades is restored.*
4 Training complete: *the balanced muscle development of the upper body holds the structures in position against gravity.*

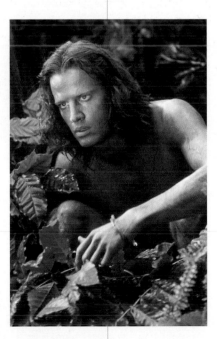

Christopher Lambert in Greystoke. *Structural fitness is part of the equipment an actor can use to develop a role.*

The bonus for me as a performer is that pilates allows me the mental space necessary to build a character. MIRANDA RICHARDSON, ACTRESS

Sports performance

Structural fitness exercises are the perfect complement to any sports performance. On an immediate level they make good warmup sequences, loosening the muscles and banishing stiffness in the joints. The breathing exercises increase oxygen supply to the brain, sharpening concentration and increasing alertness. Exercising improves coordination, which for the player of any game or sport that utilizes one arm or leg or foot, is essential to success. They also work the body in a range of movements that is essential to keep sports enthusiasts supple and mobile, helping to improve performance and prevent strains and injuries.

Skill in almost any sport tends to throw the body out of balance, just because it is always essential to concentrate on certain movements and neglect others. A qualified instructor in pilates-based structural fitness can help improve sports performance by analyzing such imbalances and their physical effects, then working out a programme of exercises to restore balance. Over the years I have occasionally been approached by professionals trained in different sports and asked to help improve performance in particular areas. I have found that the exercises can be specially adapted to improve their performance in athletics and gymnastics, and in sports such as mountaineering, golf, tennis and other racket sports, and swimming.

Amateurs can benefit as much as professionals, since pilates-based exercises help prevent damage to the body caused by trying to learn new sports techniques when the body posture is poor. For example, people often develop pain in the neck and the lower back when they take up swimming. They start with the breaststroke, and if the posture and arm and leg strokes are not learned correctly, the upper and lower spine may be damaged. Similarly, structural fitness exercises are a great preparation for winter sports. They condition the body so that lessons and practice out on the slopes are likely to be rewarding, whereas dashing off unfit for a weekend ski trip can result in an appalling shock to the body.

Structural fitness exercises can be an antidote to sports injuries. Once the break or wrench or strain has begun to heal, they can speed the healing process and prevent the distortions often caused when the body tries to compensate for the part that is temporarily out of use. It eases muscles forced into unaccustomed activity, stretches and remobilizes injured muscles, and mobilizes stiffened joints. A period off the sports field or court is a good time for taking stock of the body's overall balance

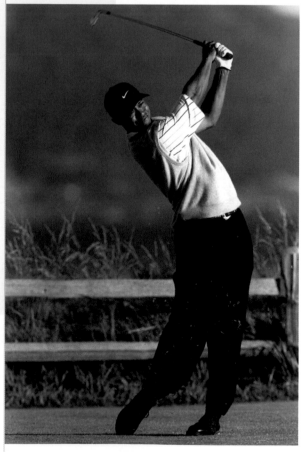

The arm sequences on page 107–08 free the upper body. They are designed to balance the upper body structures and so improve coordination. They are a great help to golf players and other sports men and women who have to wield a bat or a stick one-handed. They should be part of daily training.

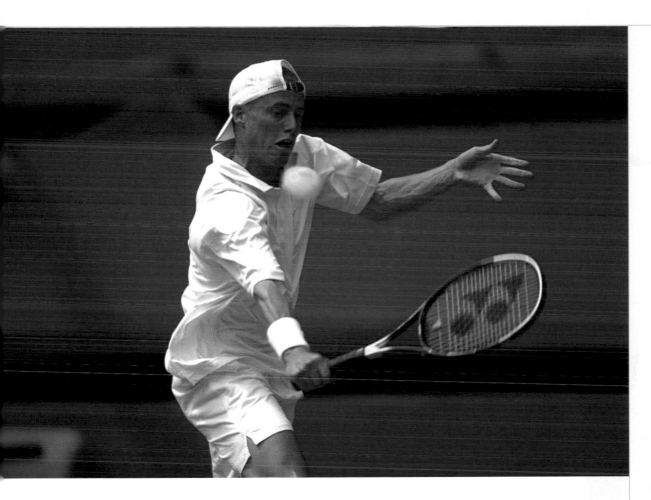

and alignment. A carefully planned fitness programme will realign the body, as well as encourage torn tendons and stretched ligaments to heal. After the injury is healed, the body may return to competition in better shape than when it left the arena.

Pronounced left or right-handed movements load undue stress on the structure of the body. Tennis players are especially susceptible because they use one hand and arm to hit the ball, generally in the same direction, and to do so they tend to position the head and neck in the same way as they anticipate hitting the ball. The weaker side has to be exercised to balance the structures of left and right sides of the body.

Pilates is the answer for everyone, especially those who suffer back and neck pain. Dreas is the maestro who never ceases to research, question, and evolve pilates to its highest level. He is my prime mentor. DR. MICHAEL DURTNALL, CONSULTANT CHIROPRACTOR

Pilates for pregnancy

Exercising during pregnancy will bring better health for mother and baby. The emphasis in structural fitness on using and strengthening the perineum – the site of episiotomies and of natural tearing during birth – could hardly serve the mother better during birth and through the postnatal period. And it does not stop there. Hoisting and carrying babies, not to mention their older brothers and sisters, if not correctly done, can result in painful misalignment, and here structural fitness routines can prevent and cure. It is essential, however, to embark on an exercise programme well before a pregnancy.

You need to look after your health and to keep fit at every stage of life. Many women only wake up to that fact when they become pregnant, but that is rather too late to begin a new fitness regime. With the exception of antenatal exercises, it is unwise to start any new exercise programme during pregnancy. I recommend that at least a year of exercising be achieved before a pregnancy, and that an exercise regime carried out through pregnancy should be planned in consultation with a qualified instructor. It is advisable to discuss the proposed regime with an obstetrician and to undergo regular monitoring.

During pregnancy an established exercise routine will need to be pared down and to change as the trimesters progress. Mothers' bodies all react differently, but it is wise to discontinue the abdominal exercises early on

(along with heavy lifting); however, squatting exercises might continue through the first trimester. After that, the cat stretch (see page 103) becomes more suitable. Leg and arm exercises should be lighter, and floor exercises cut down, since lying on the back can become more and more uncomfortable. Swimming is an excellent exercise to accompany fitness sessions, but avoid the breaststroke, which can worsen lower back problems.

Postnatal exercises are important, but it is wise to allow a few weeks for the body's hormonal balance to adjust before resuming a full exercise program after the birth. The pelvis needs time to recover from its 40-week stretch. Strenuous exercise shortly after giving birth can cause chronic back pain in the loosened joints and ligaments that tie the sacrum to the pelvic girdle.

Katherine Bucknell practises gentle strengthening exercises in the Body Conditioning Studio, using cushions and pads to support the joints of the limbs and the spine.

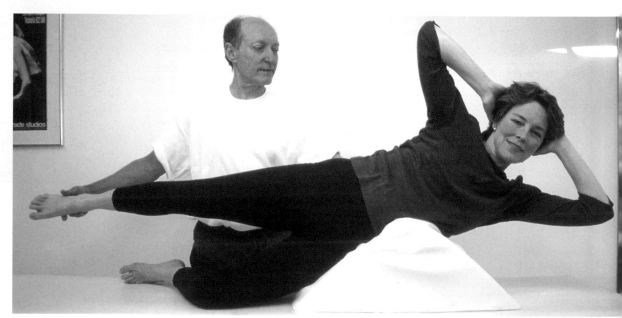

My two elder children were born when I was in my early thirties, then, after a nine-year gap, came Jack. The pregnancy alone should have flattened me, without work and the two other, very busy children. So I rested a little more, but I also exercised a little more, and a little more thoughtfully. Squash and jogging gave way to swimming, and, above all, exercise time. Both soothing and disciplining, structural fitness eased the morning sickness, buoyed my energy, and kept me mobile as my skeleton gradually came under pressure from my growing burden. The jagged-toothed sciatica I dreaded from earlier pregnancies never returned; my pelvic floor did not collapse into a tote-bag; and during the labour I stunned a few midwives by performing my favourite stretches in the hospital hallway. That and the familiar breathing to a count of six helped keep my mind off my troubles. But what surprised me most of all was that despite having prepared myself and all my household for a Victorian-style recuperation in bed while I soberly awaited my 42nd birthday, I was in fact back in regular exercise sessions when Jack was just five weeks old.

Katherine Bucknell, writer and mother

'Beware all enterprises that require new clothes', some wise person said; 'and new exercises', I would add. Pregnancy is a notoriously bad time to take up bright new skills, particularly of an athletic nature. Anyway, during both my pregnancies I did what I usually do: I took a lot of long brisk walks, and a couple of times a week I did a concentrated pilates session. For the first two trimesters this was a good routine. But towards the end of pregnancy even walking became less appealing or useful: the loosening of the joints can make you feel a bit shaky and, of course, sheer heaviness can make any walk seem steeply, miserably, uphill. (Like other women in my family, with the birth of each child I gained a full 20 kilograms (45 pounds). By contrast, the exercises really seemed to lighten the burden. And I found that I could do them, even needed to do them, with continual minor adjustments, right up until the day of the birth.

Isabel Fonseca, writer and mother

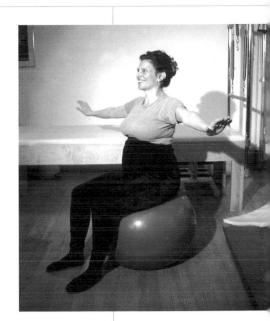

The exercise ball makes it possible to exercise aerobically but smoothly and rhythmically, without jolting the body.

Classic pilates studio apparatus is ideal for exercising during late pregnancy. Here, Dreas supervises Isabel Fonseca on the Trapeze.

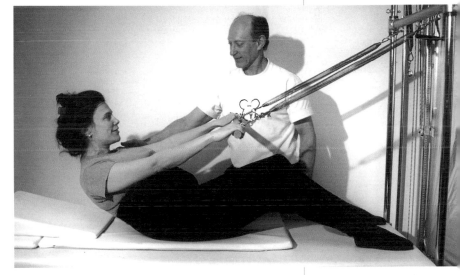

Warning

These photographs of Katherine Bucknell and Isabel Fonseca illustrate their individual fitness in examples of pilates-based structural fitness exercises. However, these exercises should not be attempted by women in any stage of pregnancy without the advice of a physician and under guidance from a fitness instructor.

Pilates from 55 to 105

At no time are the benefits of caring for the body more apparent than in later life. Eastern exercise systems, such as yoga and taiji (t'ai chi), are practised by older people. They prolong mobility and flexibility into old age and claim to maximize longevity. The West, by contrast, largely ignores exercise for older people, who are assumed to be incapable of physical improvement. Pilates-based exercises are the exception. Carefully formulated to boost circulation without straining the internal organs, and to maximize fitness without damaging body structure, pilates is the ideal exercise system for the second half of life.

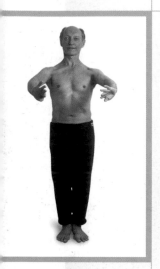

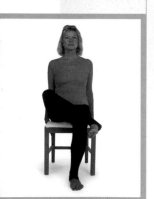

Now taking centre stage in the West is a generation of older people accustomed to a high level of physical activity, and they are transforming the image of ageing. Most enter middle age fit and active and, it is predicted, they will remain healthier, suffering less from the illnesses of ageing such as strokes and osteoporosis, incontinence and heart disease. They will remain active into old age.

But for many people who have neglected exercise, there will be obstacles to overcome. Anyone who gave up sport and exercise a decade or so ago may need to be convinced of the value of starting again. Answers to worries about imposing physical stresses on unfit bodies, about the real value of making all that effort, are found in the results of recent research. Tests carried out in the USA and elsewhere since the 1980s indicate that neglecting to use the muscles is the biggest obstacle to mobility old people face. Simple exercise tests on people over 80 who had led inactive lives in care homes for years showed that a an isotonic test (one muscle moved in one

direction) carried out over a short period can produce an improvement curve that almost hits the vertical. Ideally one should never give up exercise. But once you have done so, the body will respond if you take it up again. And so will the mind: researchers have noted improvements in alertness, memory, and interest in outside events.

However convinced they may be of the need to begin exercising again, many people will have to overcome an image problem. The impetus to exercise when older is closely related to self-image. Over time, one's image of one's body changes. People can relate to themselves as sporty and active at 16, at 26, but perhaps not at 66. The media often does not present over-50s as sporty.

Pilates exercises undermine this obstruction by gradually restoring an image of the self as that of a person who works out. While improving body structure, you unconsciously recreate an image that is real about yourself and your body. Image-restructuring begins with posture. Yet the posture to which each new individual is

If you have not exercised for years, begin with the arm circles on pages 107–08 (top). They are fun to do and they warm you up. The Sock stretch on page 148 (above) loosens the hips.

Practise simple ankle movements such as the flexion and rotation exercises on on pages 110–11 at your own speed. Practise flexing your hands and wrists in the same way (right). Strengthening the feet and ankles (far right) gives you confidence in standing and walking. Stay mobile by exercising your legs regularly.

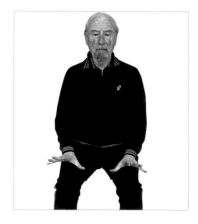

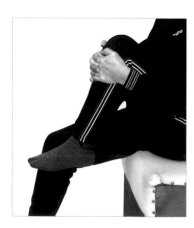

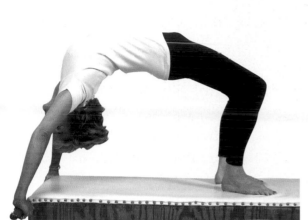

Regaining stability, balance, and flexibility bring great confidence in later life. This client approaching her sixties found that after 36 weeks of practice, she could execute a perfect backbend.

reintroduced is not static (what was once called 'deportment') but a dynamic interaction between stance and movement. Through work on posture, a trainer will seek to restore core stability and so begin to reestablish the body's normal vocabulary of movement.

The cardinal rule is not to do too much too quickly. Simple movements need to be rehearsed. The Level 1 wall exercises will help restore natural flexibility to rounded shoulders. The forward stoop so unnecessarily characteristic of old age often comes from stretching the spinal muscles and the lats. The pecs, by contrast, may be rigid, and the hip flexors are often painfully tightened.

Few exercises in this book are unsuitable for older people (but avoid hip stretches if you have had a hip replacement). If possible, begin with a class supervised by a qualified instructor who can advise about medical conditions. If you experience vertigo, improving your posture may help your circulation and revivify the structures of the inner ear responsible for balance. Level 1 wall exercises are for those who find that exercising lying down causes dizziness or discomfort. Work at your own pace, stopping if anything seems uncomfortable. Rhythm and breathing make a big contribution to the effectiveness and enjoyment of exercise.

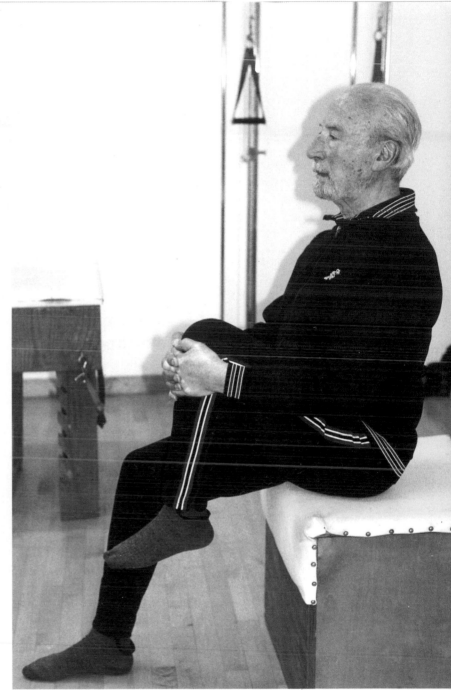

This client exercised into his nineties because it helped him keep his strength up and gave him steadiness and balance when walking. Regular practice helped him understand the benefits of moving properly: of being ever aware of maintaining good posture and relearning bad habits of movement.

I am 68 and have a back problem and various inconveniences of aging. I have benefited mentally and physically, and fully intend continuing to enjoy Dreas's dynamism. SIR IAN HOLM, FILM AND STAGE ACTOR

Useful addresses

These pages list the addresses of some organizations you can contact for information about pilates training in North America, Europe, Australia, New Zealand, and South Africa; contact numbers for suppliers of studio equipment; and the names of some notable teachers. In addition, reflecting advances in treatment for adults and children with dyslexia and other conditions related to prenatal development, I include organizations for research into neurodevelopmental delay and physical developmental integration, addressing learning difficulties, and other problems associated with dyslexia, dyspraxia, attention deficit disorder, and hyperactivity.

Pilates training

EUROPE
UK

These organizations uphold high standards of teaching to enable people to find well-qualified teachers, and ensure a common standard for teachers of pilates exercise in the UK and other European countries:

Body Control Pilates Association
17 Queensberry Mews West, London SW7 2DY
Tel: [020 7] 584 4898/Fax: [020 7] 581 2286
Information line: [0870] 169 0000 (office hours)
Pilates Foundation UK
80 Camden Road, London E17 7NF
Tel/Fax: [07071] 781 859
Alan Herdman Studios
17 Homer Row, London W1H 1HU
Tel: [020 7] 723 9953
Alan Herdman was the first person to teach pilates in London.
Body Conditioning Studio
3a Ladbroke Road, London W11
Tel: [020 7] 727 9963
Dreas Reyneke has been teaching pilates-based structural fitness since the 1970s and opened this studio in 1973. He was a founding board member of the Pilates Foundation UK and is a member today.

Austria

Gabriella Cimino, Performing Arts Studios Vienna, Zieglergasse 7, 1070 Wien
Tel: [431] 523 5656

France

Phillippe Taupin, Le Centre du Marais, 41 Rue du Temple, 75006 Paris
Tel: [331] 463 47965

Germany

Galina Rohleder
Hohenzollerndamm 158, 10713 Berlin
Tel: [49 30] 823 1124

AUSTRALIA AND NEW ZEALAND

Pilates Institute of Australasia
PO Box 1046, North Sydney,
New South Wales 2059
Tel: [612] 9267 8223/Fax: [612] 9267 8226
Net: www.pilates.net
Contact this organization for information on training, studios, and equipment in Australia and New Zealand.

Body Conditioning Studio
Suite 1, 148 Blues Point Road,
North Sydney, New South Wales 2060
Tel: [612] 9955 4588
A studio run by a well-known teacher, Penelope Latey.

NORTH AMERICA

USA

Balanced Body, Current Concepts Corp.,
7500 14th Avenue, Suite 23,
Sacramento, California 95820-3539
Tel: [916] 454 2838 & [800] 240 3539/Fax [916] 454 3120
Email: info@balancedbody.com
Net: www.balancedbody.com
Contact Ken Endelman for information about his chain of studios offering instruction in pilates-based exercise, and his excellent range of well-designed equipment.

Drago's Gym
570 West 57th St, 6th floor, New York, NY 10019
Tel: [212] 757 0724
Contact: Romana Kryzanowska
Independent teacher of pilates-based exercise, who studied under Joseph Pilates.

Kathleen S. Grant
Tish School of Art, 111 2nd Avenue,
New York, NY
Tel: [212] 998 1983
A highly respected teacher of long standing who was instructed by Joseph Pilates.

On Center Conditioning
485 E 17th Street, Suite 650, Costa Mesa, California
Tel: [714] 642 6970
Contact: Rael Jacobowitz
An independent teacher of pilates-based exercises.

The Physical-Mind Institute
1807 Second Street, #28,
Santa Fe, New Mexico 87501
Tel: [505] 988 1990]The first main body that represented pilates-based teaching in North America and Europe.

Pilates Studio
2121 Broadway, Suite 201 at 74th Street,
New York, NY 10023
Tel: [212] 875 0189
Contact: Sean P. Gallagher
A well-established New York studio.

Susanna Weiss
Tel: [718] 476 9834
A well-established teacher with a New York studio, who studied under Kathy Grant

Canada

Mary Craig
519 59th Avenue East,
Vancouver, British Columbia V5X 1Y2
Tel: [604] 324 957
An independent teacher with a studio in Vancouver.

Diana Miller
Tel: [604] 879 2900
An independent teacher with an excellent reputation, working in Vancouver.

AFRICA

South Africa

Dudley H. Tomlinson, 18 Mortimer Road,
Wynberg 7800, Cape Town
Tel: [27 21] 797 2351
One of the first studios to be set up in Africa.

Autogenics

UK

British Autogenic Society
Royal London Homeopathic Hospital, Great Ormond Street, London WC1N 3HR
Tel: [0171[713 6336
E-mail: autogenic-therapy.org.uk

Development and Learning

EUROPE

UK

The Arrow Trust
Priory Annexe, St. Mary Street, Bridgewater,
Somerset TA6 3EK
Fax: [01278] 446 261
Specializes in reading difficulties; under Dr. Colin Lane.

Institute for Neuro-Physiological Psychology [INPP]
Warwick House, 4 Stanley Place, Chester CH1 2LU
Tel/Fax [01244] 311 414
Training and research in neuro-developmental delay and reflex inhibition therapy as devised by Peter Blythe and Sally Goddard. Offers training and seminars.

Pru Miller
South West Centre, Mere, SW Wiltshire
Tel: [01747] 861330
A specialist in Developmental Integration Therapy, which may involve brushing the face or other parts of the body, who worked with Peter Blythe at the INPP.

Denmark

Dyslexia Research Laboratory
Ro/Skolovej 14 DK 3760, Gudhjem, Bornholm, Denmark
Contact: Dr. Kjeld Johansen, specialist in sound therapy.

Germany

Pedagogische Praxis,
An der Heide 1, 24235 Wendtorfer Schleuse
Contact: Thake Hansen Lauff

The Netherlands

Dutch Institute for Neuro-Physiological Psychology
Amsteldyk 138, Amsterdam
Contact: Jur Ten Hoopen

Sweden

Swedish Institute for Neuro-Physiological Psychology
Rydholmsgat, 42, S41873, Gothenberg
Contact: Catharina Johanneson Alvegard

AUSTRALIA

ANSUA – Children's Learning & Development Center
333 Given Terrace, Rosalie, Queensland
Contact: Jean Rigby

Dr. Mary Lou Shiel
80 Alexandra Street, Hunters Hill, 2110 Sydney

NORTH AMERICA

USA

Auditory Integrative Training
The Georgiana Foundation,
PO Box 2607, Westport, Connecticut 06880
Contact: Dr. Guy Berard
Specializes in sound therapy.

Autism Research Institute
4182 Adams Avenue,
San Diego, California 921169
Contact: Bernard Rimland Ph.D.

Dr. Larry Beuret, M.D.
4811 Emerson, Suite 209,
Palatine, Illinois 60067
Specialist in Neuro-Physiological Psychology.

Rolfing

EUROPE

UK

Russell Maliphant
Tel: [0171] 385 1622
E-mail: rmaliphant@compuserve.com
An independent practitioner.

Alan Rudolf
Tel: [0171] 388 6567
An independent practitioner who studied under Ida Rolf.

European Rolfing Association
Kapuziner Strasse 25, D80337,
Munich, Germany
Tel: [49] 89-543-70940

Further reading

Pilates

Friedman, Philip and Eisen, Gail. *The Pilates Method of Physical and Mental Conditioning*, Doubleday, 1980

Pilates, Joseph Hubertus. *Your Health,* Presentation Dynamics Inc., 774 Mays Blvd, Suite 10, Incline Village, NV 89451 USA, Tel: [702] 832 8210, 1998, ISBN 0-9614937-8-X

Pilates, Joseph H. and Miller, William John. *Pilate's Return to Life Through Contrology,* Presentation Dynamics, 1998

The body

Miller, Jonathan. *The Body in Question,* Pimlico Press, 1999

Hinkle, Carla Z. *Fundamentals of Anatomy and Movement,* Mosby, 1997

Thibodeau, Gary A., and Patton, Kevin T. *Structure & Function of the Body*, Mosby, 1997

Whitfield, Dr. Philip (Ed.). *The Human Body Explained,* Hamlyn/Reed Consumer Books, 1995

Exercise and movement

Gustavsen, Rolf and Streeck, Renate. *Training Therapy,* Georg Thieme Verlag, 1998

Hinkle, Carla Z. *Fundamentals of Anatomy and Movement,* Mosby, 1997

Jones, Kim & Barker, Karen. *Human Movement Explained,* Butterworth Heinemann, 1995

McArdle, William D. et al. *Exercise Physiology*, Williams & Wilkins, 1997

Shepherd, Roberta B. *Physiotherapy in Paediatrics,* Butterworth-Heinemann, 1995

Sweigard, Lulu E. *Human Movement Potential,* University Press of America, 1988

Structural fitness

Reyneke, Andreas. "Revue of the International Association for Dance Medicine and Science" published in *Dancing Times*, October 1997. (Covers the work of Marika Molnar of Westside Dance Physical Therapy, New York, Rachel-Anne Rist, Principal of the Arts Educational School, Tring, UK, and physiotherapist Craig Phillips).

Rolf, Ida P. *Rolfing,* Healing Arts Press, 1 Park Street, Rochester, Vermont 05767, ISBN 0-89281-335-0, 1989

Stirk, John L. *Structural Fitness*, Elm Tree Books, 1988, ISBN 0-241-12432-8

Thompson, Clem W. and Floyd, R.T. *Manual of Structural Kinesiology*, Mcgraw-Hill, 1997

Todd, Mabel Elsworth. *The Thinking Body,* Dance Books, 1997

Mind and body

Ashbrook, James B. (Ed.). *Brain, Culture and the Human Spirit,* University Press of America,1993

Goddard, Sally. *A Teacher's Window Into the Child's Mind, A Non-Invasive Approach to Solving Learning and Behavior Problems,* Fern Ridge Press, 1996

Keleman, Stanley. *Emotional Anatomy,* Center Press, Berkeley, 1997

Kermani, Dr. Kai. *Autogenic Training: The Effective Holistic Way to Better Health*, Souvenir Press, 1996

King, Serge. *Imagineering for Health,* Theosophical Publishing House, 1981

Miller, Pru. *A Fresh Start to Achieving True Potential,* The South West Centre, Mere, SW Wiltshire, UK, Tel 01747 861 330

General

Davis,Elizabeth. *Heart and Hands Midwives' Guide to Pregnancy and Birth,* Celestial Arts, 1998

Goodbody, John. *An Illustrated History of Gymnastics* Stanley Paul, 1982

Harvard Health Letter July 1993 *Strength Training After Sixty* (Department for Back issues, call toll free in USA: [800] 829-9045, Canada [904] 445-4662)

Kitzinger, Sheila. *The New Pregnancy and Childbirth,* Penguin, 1997

Lane, Nancy E. *The Osteoporosis Book, A Guide for Patients and their Families,* Oxford University Press, 1999

Index

Numbers in bold type (**53**) refer to a major entry and numbers in italic type (*53*) to a captioned illustration. Numbers in roman type (53) refer to a short mention in the text.

Acknowledgments

The author would like to thank:

Everyone who so generously endorsed my work, whose kind comments appear as quotations in the book and accompanying material.

Demonstrators of stances and exercises throughout the book: Bernadette Bishop, Chyna Gordon; Milena Regis; Tony Ford; page 26, Olivia Roberts; page 27 right, Jack Maguire, son of Katherine Bucknell; page 47, Russell Maliphant; page 69 bottom, Ayako Yamada; page 214, Katherine Bucknell; page 215, Isabel Fonseca; pages 216 bottom and 217 right, Milton Lomask; page 217 top, Diana Baring.
Also: pages 214–15: Ken Endelman at Balanced Body, Current Concepts Corp. for studio equipment illustrated; Debbie Moore, Pineapple Studios: exercise clothes.

All who helped me in many and various ways:
Christina Blackburn; Frances Carty; Alan Cunliffe; Dr. Michael Durtnall; Anthony Ellis; Peter Eyre; Andrew Ferguson; Dr. Barry Grimaldi; Cynthia Harvey; Marie Helvin; Graciela Kaplan; Ianthe Karanges, dance teacher; Julie Kavanagh; Gelsey Kirkland; Penelope Latey; Dr. Li Hi; Elaine MacDonald; Glynn MacDonald; Gayrie MacSween, Eileen Murphy; Jan Murray; Caro Ness; Bruce Oldfield; Priscilla and Bill Panzer; Jann Parry; Brian Peters, Maria Pietra; Patsy Pollock; Milena Regis; Clover Roope; Dr. Alan Rudolf, Master Rolfer, Dr. Iro Staebler, Nicky Searchfield, Lynn Seymour, Dudley Tomlinson; Mariela Urlezaga; Abby Ward.
And lastly, Philip Latey, Jo Levin and Liane Richards

Fiona MacIntyre at Ebury Press for this book
Fiona Roberts at Design Revolution for its design
Georgina, my agent at Capel & Land: THANK YOU

Picture credits

Every effort has been made to trace copyright holders. The publishers would be pleased to hear from anyone whose copyrights they have unwittingly infringed.

Page 10 Steve Gorton; page 13 top © I.C. Rapoport; page 14 bottom Fatimah Namder; page 16 left © I.C. Rapoport; page 17 © Landesturnverrband Sachsen-Anhalt; page 18 © I.C. Rapoport; page 20 © Science Photo Library; page 21 © The Mary Baker Eddy Library for the Betterment of Humanity, Inc; page 22 © Eye Ubiquitous/David Cumming; page 23 Chris Wilkinson Architects, Pilates Studio Design/John Donat; page 26 Fiona Roberts; page 27 top Sarah Treco; page 27 bottom © Eye Ubiquitous/Skjold; page 28 © Science Photo Library/Dr. Yorgos Nikas; page 3, © Eye Ubiquitous/Matthew McKee; page 35 © Eye Ubiquitous/Paul Seheult; page 44 Iñaki Urlezaga/Genitta; page 46 © Empics/Neal Simpson; page 47 bottom Education and Medical Illustration Services, St Bartholomew's Hospital and Medical College, London; page 55 © Empics/Mike Egerton; page 60 © Empics/Tony Marshall; page 62 © Eye Ubiquitous/James Mollison 1995; page 67 © Eye Ubiquitous/Paul Seheult; page 69 © Empics/Adam Davy; page 70 © Empics/Phil O'Brien; page 71 © Empics/Tony Marshall; page 78, Eye Ubiquitous/Steve Miller; page 115 © Getty One/Image Bank; page 125, Iñaki Urlezaga/Genitta; page 147, Iñaki Urlezaga/Genitta; page 157, Iñaki Urlezaga/Genitta; page 201 © Empics/S&G; page 207 centre, Fatimah Namder; page 208 © Powerstock; page 209, Dr. Michael Durtnall/Cliff Barden Photography; page 210 left & right © The Ronald Grant Archive; page 211 top, Dreas Reyneke; page 211 bottom © The Ronald Grant Archive; page 212 © Empics/Tony Marshall; page 213 Empics/Jon Buckle; pages 214 and 215, Fatimah Namder; page 216 bottom and 217, Dreas Reyneke

Dreas Reyneke bears witness to his position in the pilates movement: one of the best half dozen in the world. This book will benefit practitioners new and old.

TERENCE STAMP, FILM ACTOR AND WRITER